About Island Press

Since 1984, the nonprofit organization Island Press has been stimulating, shaping, and communicating ideas that are essential for solving environmental problems worldwide. With more than 1,000 titles in print and some 30 new releases each year, we are the nation's leading publisher on environmental issues. We identify innovative thinkers and emerging trends in the environmental field. We work with world-renowned experts and authors to develop cross-disciplinary solutions to environmental challenges.

Island Press designs and executes educational campaigns, in conjunction with our authors, to communicate their critical messages in print, in person, and online using the latest technologies, innovative programs, and the media. Our goal is to reach targeted audiences—scientists, policy makers, environmental advocates, urban planners, the media, and concerned citizens—with information that can be used to create the framework for long-term ecological health and human well-being.

Island Press gratefully acknowledges major support from The Bobolink Foundation, Caldera Foundation, The Curtis and Edith Munson Foundation, The Forrest C. and Frances H. Lattner Foundation, The JPB Foundation, The Kresge Foundation, The Summit Charitable Foundation, Inc., and many other generous organizations and individuals.

The opinions expressed in this book are those of the author(s) and do not necessarily reflect the views of our supporters.

Reinventing Food Banks
and Pantries

Reinventing Food Banks and Pantries

NEW TOOLS TO END HUNGER

Katie S. Martin

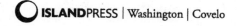

ISLANDPRESS | Washington | Covelo

Library of Congress Control Number: 2020944714

All Island Press books are printed on environmentally responsible materials.

Manufactured in the United States of America
10 9 8 7 6

Keywords: charitable food, client choice, diabetes prevention, emergency food, food assistance, food hubs, food pantry, food security, hunger, hunger-relief organizations, job training, nutrition education, SNAP, working poor, wraparound services

To Chris,
Thank you for sharing this vision and journey with me.
You make me a better person and you made this book
better with your thoughtful suggestions.

Contents

Preface   xi

1. Introduction   1
2. History of Food Assistance Programs   16
3. A Paradigm Shift in How We Talk about Hunger   36
4. A Welcoming Culture   56
5. The Dignity of Choice   73
6. Promotion of Healthy Food   90
7. Connection to Community Services   114
8. The Vital Role of Volunteers   135
9. Evaluation: What Gets Measured Gets Done   152
10. Structural Inequalities and Systems Change   176
11. Equity within Food Banks and Pantries   198
12. New Partners and Community Food Hubs   216
13. Conclusion: Take One Step   239

About the Author   255

Preface

The director of the Kelly Memorial Food Pantry in El Paso, Texas, was seeing the same clients come routinely to the pantry and was looking for a new approach to help families in more meaningful ways. She heard about an innovative food pantry called Freshplace in Hartford, Connecticut, and the board of directors reached out to me to learn more. I started collaborating with the wonderful staff, board of directors, and volunteers at Kelly Memorial to describe a different approach to treating the problem of hunger.

I described a paradigm shift away from the traditional model of handing people a bag of food to allowing clients to choose their food with dignity. I helped train coaches to provide motivation and help clients set goals for becoming food secure and self-sufficient so they wouldn't need to keep coming to get food at the pantry. I suggested ways to design their pantry to be an empowering place to provide more than just food.

The team was ready and started to make changes. They transformed the look of their pantry with a huge welcome sign, a client choice pantry, a resource center with computers and space for coaching, and additional classes. They revamped their programming to offer individualized coaching and wraparound services. They recently renamed their pantry the Kelly Center for Hunger Relief and they call their program Fresh Start. Over the course of the past few years, they have also transformed many lives. They celebrate accomplishments of their members with graduation ceremonies. One of the first graduates explained, "This program not only has the heart and humility of supporting and motivating members to have a 'Fresh Start,' more important, they guide you with love while helping you put your desires and goals of life in order. They connect you with the many services that you need for your own personal growth."

I have seen multiple food pantries make these types of comprehensive changes and the positive impact they have had on people's lives. This type of transformative food pantry is entirely possible but not common. My motivation for writing this book is to share examples of a holistic approach to hunger, the lessons I've learned, and practical tools to help you implement these changes in your community so we can help more people not only to be food secure but to thrive.

The Role of Food Banks and Food Pantries

For many years at Foodshare, the regional food bank where I work in Greater Hartford, Connecticut, our motto was, "When hunger stops, so will we." This was intended to be inspirational and achievable, because food banks were created to be short-term, to treat an emergency situation, and then to end. Food banks were never intended to be long-term solutions. But over the past forty years, rather than closing our doors, food banks have become institutional pillars in local communities around the country. Food banks and food pantries are essential services when people fall on hard times. Foodshare's new motto is, "Hunger is big. Our community is bigger." We recognize that it takes a community approach to tackle hunger. Our tagline is, "We're changing what it means to be a food bank." Imagine what that can look like.

Some people say that we should put food banks out of business and that food pantries are not the answer to hunger. Many have argued that the charitable food system takes the government off the hook from providing a strong and stable safety net. I understand this argument. I agree that food banks are a stark example of how our government has failed. We absolutely need a stronger and more secure federal safety net, starting with livable wages and including federal food assistance programs, affordable housing, health care, and child care.

But here's the thing. I think those of us in the charitable food system of food banks and food pantries took ourselves off the hook too. For many years, we stood on the sidelines of policy debates and didn't pressure the government to strengthen the social safety net. For many years, we served more people, distributed more pounds of food, built bigger warehouses, and focused on feeding people today. But change is happening. Food banks and food pantries around the country are promoting equity, creating nutrition policies, advocating for federal nutrition programs, and developing paths to stability. I want to be part of the change. How about you?

Imagine the systemic changes we can make to promote health and financial well-being, and reduce stigma and inequities, when we collectively work together.

Let's harness the amazing energy, talent, resources, and goodwill of this massive national network. Imagine the systemic changes we can make to promote health and financial well-being, and reduce stigma and inequities, when we collectively work together.

My Background

In 1994, I accepted a summer internship at the Food Bank For New York City. I worked as a food bank monitor, and I visited over one hundred food pantries, soup kitchens, and shelters to make sure they were abiding by the food bank rules. I traveled through all five boroughs of the city, rode almost every subway and bus line in the city, and saw more sections of the city than many native New Yorkers. It was quite a learning experience to witness people lined up for bags of food in trash-strewn neighborhoods in the South Bronx and in tree-lined neighborhoods in Manhattan. I spoke with many food pantry directors and with many food pantry clients about their experiences dealing with food insecurity.

I have a vivid memory of visiting a food pantry in lower Manhattan on a beautiful Friday morning, with ample sunshine and a bright blue sky. The beauty of the day was spoiled by the fact that dozens of people were lined up, wrapping around a corner, waiting to receive food. They slowly moved toward the front of the line until eventually being handed a bag of food. Volunteers would pass bags up the steps from a hatch door in the basement where the food was stored. It wasn't glamorous, and it definitely didn't feel like picking up food at a grocery store. This scene would replay again the following week, and the week after. That summer, I realized that handing out food is not enough; we need more holistic approaches to the problem of hunger.

Throughout my career, I have interviewed hundreds of people who have experienced food insecurity and asked about their coping strategies and their opinions about food pantries. I have seen firsthand what poverty and hunger look like. I have sat on mattresses in living rooms that served as bedrooms, people have shown me their empty refrigerators, and parents have described their anxiety about getting enough food for their families. I have witnessed hunger in Connecticut, one of the wealthiest states in America. These experiences fueled my commitment to understand the problem and its root causes and to try to develop long-term solutions.

For the past decade I have collaborated closely with Feeding America, and multiple food banks and food pantries around the country. In 2018 I began working at Foodshare, the regional food bank of Greater Hartford, Connecticut. Being "on the inside" of a food bank gives me firsthand knowledge of the complex operations involved with collecting and distributing charitable food and a clearer understanding of the challenges and opportunities we face as a national charitable food system.

It is time to shift our focus from an emergency response toward empowerment and from short-term transactions of food to long-term transformations of lives.

But First, Gratitude

Throughout this book, I may seem critical of our charitable food system. I will point out flaws, I will challenge the status quo, and I will argue for change. But please don't mistake this for disrespect. I have a huge amount of admiration for the incredibly caring and hardworking people who address the problem of hunger in their communities. Who collect food from wholesalers and grocery stores and distribute to those who don't have enough. Who have developed creative solutions, often on shoe-string budgets with mostly volunteer staffs. I wouldn't have decided to join a food bank if I didn't believe in the value of this work. In fact, my hope is that many of you are part of this dedicated group: directors and volunteers of food banks and food pantries who have committed your time, talent, and ideas to the job of tackling hunger. Thank you for all you do!

We are doing very good work in the charitable food system. I don't want to diminish the incredible efforts we have made to address hunger. I want to honor that good work. But (you knew there was a but) we can do better. We can recognize that food alone won't solve the problem. It is time to shift our focus from an emergency response toward empowerment and from short-term transactions of food to long-term transformations of lives.

It is important to recognize our limitations and flaws, not simply to criticize, but to highlight opportunities for growth. I am an optimist by nature. We have a strong network of food banks nationwide, and I am heartened by what we can accomplish. I think sometimes we set our sights too low, and I will encourage you to dream bigger. I will provide data and stories about the challenges and complexity of food insecurity, but this book is not just about the problem. It is about strategies that you can act upon. This book focuses on solutions for creating a healthier and more holistic way to address food insecurity. I don't have all the answers, and there is no silver bullet to solve the problem of hunger. But there are many things we can do to tackle the problem differently.

I believe many of you are ready for a change. We have a robust national network of charitable food banks and food pantries that are primed for new approaches, new leaders, and a new way of thinking. Many people are planning to start a food pantry from scratch and are looking for guidance. We have an amazing foundation to build upon and a network of incredibly thoughtful, smart, and caring individuals who can lead the way. Including you.

A Calling

In many ways, I think of my work as more of a calling than simply a career. One of my core beliefs is that we all have unique talents, and it is part of our responsibility in life to recognize our gifts and share them with the world. As Pablo Picasso once said, "The meaning of life is to find your gift. The purpose of life is to give it away." Throughout my life, I believe God has been calling me to do this work and to share my experiences. I know many of you choose to work in, volunteer with, or donate to antihunger programs because of your faith. Others are called by personal ethics or experiences with hunger. Whatever your motivation to be of service, I hope you will heed the call to make an impact in your community.

I welcome you to join the movement to change the way we think about and address the problem of hunger. Tackling hunger is about ensuring that people not only have enough food but have the opportunity to share their beautiful, unique gifts with the rest of the world. Imagine how much ingenuity is lost because millions of our neighbors are focused on making sure they have enough food rather than developing their talents.

Mentors

In the movie *The Commitments*, the lead character wants to start a band. When he interviews potential band members, the first question he asks is "Who are your influences?" The people who influence our work say a lot about who we are and how we view the world. Many people have influenced me, provided mentorship, inspired me, and paved the way for me to write this book.

First and foremost, Tony Hall. I'm not sure if I would be doing antihunger work today if it weren't for my summer internship with Congressman Tony P. Hall from my hometown of Dayton, Ohio. In the summer of 1990, I worked for Congressman Hall in his Washington, DC, office in the Rayburn Building. I was inspired by his commitment to alleviate hunger both domestically and internationally, and this informed my choice of graduate school and future career path. Young adults and parents out there, never underestimate the power of a summer internship (even unpaid) to shape the direction of a life. Tony Hall is an ambassador for antihunger work globally, and recently he created the Hall Hunger Initiative to focus work back in Dayton.

Wanting to combine my undergraduate degree in political science with my new focus on hunger, I found a fabulous graduate program at Tufts University in the Friedman School of Nutrition Science and Policy. What really drew me to the school was the Center on Hunger, Poverty, and Nutrition Policy, directed by Dr. Larry Brown. I received terrific training and advisement from Drs. Larry Brown, John Cook, and Bea Rogers, as well as other great faculty at Tufts, who taught me about the important connection between nutritional science and policy change to ensure food security.

As a young researcher, I learned a lot about the charitable food system from Jan Poppendieck and her inspirational and influential book *Sweet Charity?*, which is still relevant many years later. I was fortunate to work with Mark Winne at the Hartford Food System while I completed my doctorate. Mark is the author of four books, including *Closing the Food Gap*, and a visionary who isn't afraid to question the status quo and argue for meaningful change in our food system. Mark also introduced me to the wonderful staff at Island Press, who decided to publish this book, so I will be forever grateful. Speaking of Island Press, thank you to the thoughtful team of marketing staff and editors, especially Emily Turner who helped me throughout the process of publishing my first book.

More recently, I have been inspired by Nick Saul and his pioneering work at The Stop in Toronto, Canada. I stopped using a highlighter while reading his book *The Stop*, because every page was turning yellow. Nick's holistic approach to food security, good food, and advocacy helped lead to the development of Community Food Centres Canada, for which the goal is to build health, belonging, and social justice in low-income communities through the power of food.

Over the past few years, I've been influenced by Jen Sincero and her best-selling book *You Are a Badass: How to Stop Doubting Your Greatness and Start Living an Awesome Life* (that is absolutely the full title!). Jen writes in a hilarious way about living your life to its fullest, about setting goals, and achieving your dreams. I encourage you all to be a badass to make changes in the charitable food system.

I include these books at the ends of chapters, and if you haven't read them, I strongly encourage you to because they will inform, inspire, and influence you to think differently and dream bigger. The world needs more visionary and action-oriented people to do this important work!

To my colleague Dr. Jessica Sanderson from Urban Alliance, I have learned a lot from you about motivational interviewing, trauma-informed care, and practical ways to provide coaching in food pantries, and I value your insight. To my colleague and friend Dr. Marlene Schwartz, who directs the University of Connecticut Rudd Center for Food Policy and Obesity, thanks for being a great partner to help develop and evaluate the SWAP stoplight nutrition system for food banks and food pantries. To my Simsbury squad—you know who you are—thanks for having my back and always making me laugh.

My mom and dad were my earliest mentors and were role models for how to serve others through their careers, my dad as a psychologist and my mom as a nurse. Thanks for your continuous support and love! To my sisters, Bridgette, Sheila, and Kelly, and my cousin Mary—you are all rock stars, and you inspire me to be a badass! To my kids Carson and Brian, and my host son Kenny (Kehinde), you add so much joy to my life, and I am proud to be your mom!

And the biggest cheerleader for me writing this book is my husband of twenty-five years, my best friend, Chris Drew. Thank you for nudging, encouraging, and supporting me every step of the way!

Action Steps

- Be curious. Ask questions.
- Think about your unique gifts and heed the call to make an impact in your community.
- Keep an open mind about the role of food banks and food pantries and how they can evolve.
- Take an honest look at the way your local programs are operated and designed.

Resources

Poppendieck, Janet. *Sweet Charity? Emergency Food and the End of Entitlement*. New York: Viking Press, 1998.

Saul, Nick, and Andrea Curtis. *The Stop: How the Fight for Good Food Transformed a Community and Inspired a Movement*. Brooklyn, NY: Melville House, 2013.

Sincero, Jen. *You Are a Badass: How to Stop Doubting Your Greatness and Start Living an Awesome Life*. Philadelphia: Running Press, 2013.

Winne, Mark. *Closing the Food Gap: Resetting the Table in the Land of Plenty*. Boston: Beacon Press, 2008.

CHAPTER 1
Introduction

Imagine that your neighbor Maria just lost her job. She had a couple months' worth of savings, but soon she is having a hard time paying all of the bills. When she realizes that she won't have enough food to feed her kids by the end of the week, she decides to ask for help. She heard about a local food pantry in town, and she decides to park her pride at the curb and check it out.

Imagine that as she walks in a woman greets her warmly and asks if she's been to the pantry before. Maria ducks her head and says no. The woman welcomes her and explains that she came to the pantry for the first time not long ago herself. The woman introduces Maria to a volunteer who will help her shop in the pantry. The volunteer hands Maria a small shopping cart, and Maria almost feels like she's at the grocery store. Since it is Maria's first time, the volunteer explains that the mission of the pantry is to be a community hub where guests come for food, connection, and much more.

The volunteer points out signs on the pantry shelves for how many food items to take, and she encourages Maria to choose the food she wants. Imagine that there is a table with recipes and another table with freshly brewed coffee and water. Last year the doctor told Maria that she is prediabetic, and Maria is pleasantly surprised to see signs showing which foods are diabetes friendly. As she walks down the aisles, she picks out food that she knows her kids will like. Imagine that there is a glass-front refrigerator displaying fruit, milk, and yogurt. Her daughter is going to love the yogurt! Imagine that there is also a shelf filled with diapers, soap, toilet paper, and laundry detergent. It's summertime and the pantry received a lot of squash, so the volunteer tells Maria to take as much as she likes.

Imagine that as she shops, Maria sees a neighbor that she knows from her daughter's school. She says hi and asks if Maria is coming to the resource fair that's being held at the pantry later in the week. Maria asks her about the fair. The friend explains that different community agencies and local businesses come once a month to describe their programs and services for people who shop at the pantry. It's an easy way to learn about resources in the community and to enroll in different programs. The neighbor encourages Maria to come and check it out. Maria had no idea that the food pantry offered these types of services. She thought the pantry just provided food.

Imagine that the pantry is bustling with a steady flow of activity as guests and volunteers interact. One of the volunteers explains that guests can come to the pantry once a week, and in addition to the food, the pantry offers classes and workshops. The volunteer says her favorite is the yoga class that helps to keep her stress down. She points to a large white board with information and sign-up sheets. There is a job training program, diabetes prevention, computer class, and advocacy 101. She explains that the pantry also has a coach that is available to provide one-on-one support to help guests work on goals.

Imagine that when Maria drove to the pantry, she felt a wave of embarrassment wash over her because she never thought she would need to ask for charity. When she walks out of the pantry, she feels encouraged and empowered. Imagine that Maria goes to the resource fair, she starts going to some of the classes, and she meets regularly with a coach to work on budgeting and applying for a new job. She takes a diabetes prevention class, is eating more vegetables, and brings her blood sugar down. After three months, she starts a new job, and now she comes to the pantry to volunteer. Maria met some new friends at the pantry and she is becoming an advocate for her community.

Can you imagine this type of food pantry? Do you have a pantry like this in your community? I hope so. This book will provide tools and resources for creating this type of holistic, empowering, healthy, community food hub. The type of food pantry that provides food but also serves as a springboard for stability, food security, and well-being so people won't need to rely on the food pantry long-term.

Hungry for Change

Many people I have met, who either receive food from food pantries or who work at food pantries and food banks, are looking for new solutions beyond bags of food. They are hungry for change. Despite the fact that hunger is a chronic problem that affected one out of every nine Americans in 2018, it is preventable. We are a nation of very smart, caring, and innovative people. So why is it that millions of Americans do not have enough food to eat?

In the United States, we have built an impressive network of food banks that have grown in number and size over five decades. According to Food Bank News, at least 370 food banks across the United States acquire perishable and nonperishable food and redistribute it to organizations that provide food directly to individuals. There are over 60,000 hunger-relief organizations such as food pantries and community kitchens in the United States. They operate in virtually every community around the country. Feeding America is the largest hunger-relief organization in the United States, serves a nationwide network of 200 food banks, and is the second largest charity in the United States.

That we have such pervasive food insecurity is not because we do not have enough food.

The focus of this national network has been, and continues to be, to tackle hunger by providing more food to more people. We've done a great job of that. Collectively in 2018, the Feeding America network distributed over 4 billion meals (with a *b*) to people in need.

Yet, if this tactic were successful, we would have solved the problem of hunger a long time ago. Sadly, food insecurity remains a persistent public health problem, affecting over 37 million Americans in 2018. Millions of our neighbors worry about having enough food at the end of the week or the end of the month. That we have such pervasive food insecurity is not because we do not have enough food. We lack justice and equity within our food system, we lack the courage or patience to tackle the root causes of poverty, and we lack the political will to ensure living wages and a strong social safety net. We can do better.

It is time for a new approach. Most food banks have been operating for over thirty-five years, and there is a new wave of leaders who are coming into the network with fresh ideas and solutions. Maybe you are one of these new leaders—welcome to the network! At the same time, many local food pantry directors are nearing retirement, and we will need a new generation of leaders to take their place. Maybe you are thinking of a new career path and can help pave a new direction. Community colleges, health clinics, and hospitals are starting new food pantries within their facilities. Rather than maintaining the status quo, we have an opportunity (and, I believe, a responsibility) to reinvent what food banks and food pantries look like and how they operate.

In an effort to provide "emergency" food, we have designed systems that are largely transactional, with a focus on serving as many people as possible as quickly as possible. I provide a roadmap for designing food pantries that are instead relational and can be transformational, and which emphasize health, social justice, community, and a person-centered design.

My hope is this book will inspire you to think differently about why hunger exists and how we have responded to it, with both public and private programs. This book provides tools to create a healthier and more comprehensive approach to address food insecurity. Throughout, I give examples of best practices and model food pantries. I suggest different options for incorporating these concepts in your own programs. I'm impatient by nature. Don't worry, I won't make you wait until the last chapter to give you a few solutions. At the end of every chapter, I provide action steps that you can take today in your community.

Please do not see these strategies as one-size-fits-all or all-or-nothing. I encourage you to think of the following pages as a menu.

Here is my appeal as you consider the various tools outlined in this book. Please do not see these strategies as one-size-fits-all or all-or-nothing. I encourage you to think of the following pages as a menu. If you find one idea that appeals to you and you decide to implement it in your food bank or food pantry, terrific! Maybe you decide to try three new ideas, like an appetizer, entrée, and dessert—that's wonderful! You can start small and take one bite.

Upcoming Chapters

Here is a look ahead and what you can expect from this book. In chapter 2, I provide a brief history of food assistance programs in the United States, starting with food stamps and child nutrition programs. After examining how food banks and food pantries developed, we'll look at an example of a holistic food pantry model that offers connection, coaching, and more than just food. In chapter 3, I describe key terms used throughout the book and make suggestions for new language to describe our work.

In chapter 4, I encourage you to think about the experience of clients (which I will often refer to as guests or customers) when they go to a food pantry. I offer examples of how to design pantries to create a welcoming environment with attention to seating and signage, how to designate a greeter, and how to de-escalate situations when tensions arise. To help move food pantries from transactional to transformational, we can train staff and volunteers in hospitality and customer service, taking tips from the retail and hotel industries.

In chapter 5, I detail how to switch from a traditional food pantry model where volunteers prebag food and hand food to clients, to a client choice model in which the pantry is designed like a grocery store where clients can shop for their food with dignity. When volunteers spend less of their time bagging food, they can spend more time greeting guests and building relationships.

In chapter 6, I describe the strong connection between hunger and health and why we should focus not just on pounds of food but on the nutritional quality of the food. If you are on a limited budget in a low-income community, it is easy to access and afford highly processed food such as soda, ramen noodles, and chips, which contribute to chronic diseases. We can use a lens of social justice to help level the playing field by making it easier for guests to access fresh fruits, vegetables, and lean protein in food pantries. I provide examples for promoting healthy food at food banks and food pantries, including a stoplight nutrition ranking system and tools for asking food donors to donate healthier food.

In chapter 7, I highlight the importance of building relationships between guests and staff to address the root causes of hunger. I describe an evidence-based program called More Than Food. After providing billions of meals to people over decades, we know that it takes more than food to end hunger. Food pantries that offer More Than Food have coaches who are trained in motivational interviewing skills in a strength-based and nonjudgmental approach to meet people where they are. The coaches work one-on-one with individuals to identify the reasons why the family is struggling with food insecurity and to connect the family with community resources that will build their self-sufficiency, such as job training, skill building, and education.

The charitable food system would not exist if it weren't for the valuable contributions of volunteers, which we'll discuss in chapter 8. In chapter 9, I describe the importance of conducting research to evaluate how we're doing and to measure the impact of our programs on the people we serve.

In chapter 10, I explore the underlying reasons why people struggle to get enough food, including income inequality, structural racism, and systemic injustices that create and perpetuate food insecurity for marginalized groups. We will talk about the working poor and strategies for creating bridges out of poverty. Recognizing the root causes of hunger can help us advocate for a stronger social safety net and living wages.

If we want to advocate for policy change outside our organizations, it is important to look within. In chapter 11, I describe examples for building equity, diversity, and inclusion within food banks and food pantries and how to include the voices of those who have experienced hunger. Sharing the stories and experiences of the people who visit food pantries can help reduce social stigma and serve as a powerful advocacy tool.

New organizations are interested in partnering with food banks and food pantries, which I describe in chapter 12. For example, health-care providers and colleges recognize that their patients and students may be struggling with food insecurity and are finding creative ways to increase access to healthy food and reduce health disparities. The tools and action steps throughout the book should be helpful for new organizations that are just getting started and may not have thought about how to design or run a food pantry. In chapter 12, I also provide suggestions for putting these tools together in a holistic community food hub like the one that Maria visited in the beginning of this chapter.

In chapter 13, I provide tools for building organizational buy-in to adopt these new approaches in food banks and food pantries. Throughout the book I show examples of programs and organizations that are making substantial impacts and can serve as role models for others. I am partnering with Feeding America, multiple food banks, and food pantries, and I highlight best practices. We don't have to start from scratch or re-create the wheel. We can work within the existing and robust system of food banks, food pantries, and community kitchens blanketing our communities. This book offers tangible action steps for operating food pantries that will promote the health and stability of families and create a bridge for self-sufficiency rather than merely a short-term Band-Aid of food.

Reinvention of the Charitable Food System

My goal for this book is bold yet simple: to reinvent the way we provide charitable food in America. We can improve the quality of the food provided, the design of our food pantries, the language we use to describe our work, the way we treat and greet people when they arrive, our methods of measuring success, and, ultimately, the long-term solutions to hunger. To reinvent a whole system that has developed over multiple decades is a big goal. I know that sounds lofty, and maybe unrealistic, arrogant, naïve, or even crazy.

But think about it—there are 200 food banks in the Feeding America network and over 60,000 community programs providing charitable food nationwide. This massive network includes staff, volunteers, food donors, boards of directors, and financial donors. Food banks and food pantries are in every community in America, and since you're reading this, then you're probably involved with one as an employee, volunteer, or donor.

Change won't happen overnight. The re-invention I am describing will come with small steps taken by many individuals. In many ways, food banks and food pantries are already reinventing themselves. I describe many innovative approaches and creative solutions already taking place around the country. I can tell you, there is interest and momentum for these changes. The wind is at our back!

My goal for this book is bold yet simple: to reinvent the way we provide charitable food in America.

Reinvention requires imagination. It requires thinking outside the box, trying new approaches, and being creative. It means getting out of our comfort zones, failing, learning about what didn't work, and trying again. It is a process of continual revision and evolution. To quote John Lennon from his classic song "Imagine," "You may say I'm a dreamer, but I'm not the only one." To end hunger, we need many dreamers. I hope you'll join me. Imagine what our charitable food system can look like.

Long-term Vision

This chapter opened with my vision of a community food hub. Throughout the book, you will read about how we can create these kinds of organizations as part of a holistic and just charitable food system. Here is a quick preview.

Food banks will play a leadership role in building the capacity of their network of food programs and coordinating services between agencies.

The goal is to provide both healthy food to those in need and wraparound services so people won't need to use the pantry long-term. Over time, we want to create community food hubs as anchor organizations that are open several days a week with some evening and weekend hours and staffed with full-time employees paid living wages with benefits. These food hubs will offer healthy food, including fresh produce, along with nutrition education and health promotion, to help reduce health disparities.

These holistic food hubs will have resource centers to provide services beyond food. Trained coaches will offer wraparound services, helping guests enroll in federal food assistance programs and community programs to address the root causes of hunger. They will provide a welcoming and empowering space for guests that is not stigmatizing. They will be designed as one-stop shopping sites where local community organizations come to describe services, enroll people in programs, and offer classes on-site. Food hubs will serve as community spaces where guests can advocate for bigger systems and policy changes, raise their voices about their experience with food insecurity, and help develop long-term solutions. Guests won't feel embarrassed to go get help. Local, state, and, eventually, federal government will help fund the community food hubs as part of a robust safety net to provide basic needs of food and a bridge to help people get back on their feet. The tools throughout this book will help you create this vision in your community.

Intended Audience

My intended audience for this book is primarily people working at food banks and food pantries—you will be familiar with the key concepts and have a direct stake in this work. This book is also meant to appeal to a broader audience because it will take a lot of people to reinvent the charitable food system, for example:

- Volunteers, including boards of directors;
- Food donors;
- Financial donors, including corporations and foundations;
- Antihunger and antipoverty organizations;
- Academic researchers;
- Community organizers;
- Nutrition professionals;
- Health-care and social service providers; and
- Policy makers at the town, state, and federal levels.

There are opportunities for each of you to get involved and be part of this movement. We need your diverse expertise and talent.

What This Book Is Not About

To set expectations, let me describe what this book is *not* about. Other books have been written about federal food assistance programs, such as the Supplemental Nutrition Assistance Program (SNAP, formerly called food stamps) and the National School Lunch Program. These programs serve as the foundation of the government's response to food insecurity. They are the first line of defense against hunger. I will mention opportunities to support and provide outreach for federal food assistance, but that is not the focus of this book.

Other books have been written about the broader community food system, including farmers markets, community gardens, and local initiatives to increase access to local, healthy food. Several books have focused on food policies and the impact they have on nutrition standards, food prices, and food marketing. Recent books have also focused on food waste and the environmental consequences of our food production and consumption. At the end of each chapter I provide resources and suggested reading, including many of these terrific books, but I won't emphasize those topics.

This book is specifically about improving our charitable food system: building the capacity of food banks and pantries to tackle hunger with a more holistic and long-term approach. In my opinion, there is a gap in the literature on this subject, and I hope to contribute to this specific field of work.

For most of my career I worked at a university, and much of my writing has been intended for academic audiences, which involves detailed citations to reference all sources of information and to carefully document previous literature on a subject matter. As you can tell, that is not the style of this book. I want this book to be more conversational. You're welcome.

The New Normal

I am writing this book during the unprecedented Coronavirus (COVID-19) pandemic health crisis in the spring of 2020. The role of our charitable food system becomes even more apparent when we are faced with this type of emergency. The COVID-19 crisis underscores the essential service provided by food banks and food pantries to respond to the basic need for food. In many ways, the food banking system is built to respond to emergencies just like this—we have the infrastructure of staff, trucks, and warehouses to act quickly to pick up and deliver food throughout our community.

We are in business to provide food when people fall on hard times. And wow, are these hard times! Food banks and food pantries are adjusting to the new reality with new types of delivery systems, such as drive-through food distributions to enforce social distancing. Food banks are responding to fluctuations in food donations and showing how nimble and flexible we can be because we are accustomed to an ever-changing supply of donated food.

But this crisis also exposes cracks and vulnerabilities in our system. Charitable food relies heavily on volunteers, many of whom are senior citizens and need to stay home to avoid exposure to the virus. Food pantries often do not collaborate with one another,

But this crisis also exposes cracks and vulnerabilities in our system.

and many are open limited hours, making it hard for people seeking help to easily receive it.

More importantly, COVID-19 underscores structural inequalities in our society and the reality that millions of Americans are living paycheck to paycheck. It has become clear that people of color face a triple threat of being more at risk for food insecurity, more likely to lose their jobs during COVID-19, and more susceptible to the disease. It's important to remember that before COVID-19, over 37 million households were already struggling to get enough food.

In response to COVID-19, the government didn't just sit back and applaud the charitable food system. They stepped up like governments need to do to provide for basic needs. Owing to the hardship caused by many businesses closing and people being newly out of work, the federal government responded. They provided direct payments through stimulus checks, suspended student loan payments, waived restrictions and increased benefits for SNAP, and streamlined unemployment benefits. Congress passed the bipartisan Families First Coronavirus Response Act, which requires certain employers to provide employees with paid family and medical leave. This type of government response is what antipoverty and antihunger advocates have been calling for, for decades.

The charitable food system cannot solve the problem of hunger alone. Government at various levels (local, state, federal) must be the key driver to end hunger through progressive policies such as a livable wage, affordable health care, paid sick and family leave, free and

Rather than being apolitical, food banks can use their tremendous platforms to advocate for robust policy changes.

reduced-price meals for children, and SNAP benefits. Rather than being apolitical, food banks can use their tremendous platforms to advocate for robust policy changes. Food pantries can create opportunities for people who have experienced hunger to speak up about injustices that hinder the health and well-being of their community.

As we advocate for broader social changes, we can also make important changes to our own food banks and pantries today. My hope is that once we emerge from sheltering in place and start to create our new normal, we will use this as an opportunity to shift from basic emergency services to advanced best practices. We have an opportunity not only to rebuild but to reinvent the way we provide services. After COVID-19, we will no longer be able to say "this is how we've always done things." It is absolutely possible, and necessary, to evolve and make changes. This book will give you some ideas for how to start.

Each food bank has its unique mission statement, host of programs, and strategic goals. Each food pantry has its own unique layout, hours of operation, and crew of volunteers. Each local community has its own strengths, challenges, and approach. There is not a cookie-cutter, one-size-fits-all solution to tackling hunger. Yet we can learn from one another. Unlike federal food assistance programs like SNAP or the School Lunch Program, which are highly standardized and regulated, the charitable food system is grass roots and independently run. While this creates challenges in terms of sharing information and standardizing services, it also provides a great deal of flexibility and allows for innovation to solve the problem. It allows each of us to make changes in our local communities and within our programs, without waiting for a policy change or mandate from the federal government. We can start now.

Ready to learn more? Let's get started. . .

Action Steps

- Think about how your local community was impacted by COVID-19 and how you adapted your services.
- Be open to new ideas.
- Identify programs or approaches to providing food that need to be restructured after COVID-19.
- Set a goal to make at least one change.

Resources

Berg, Joel. *All You Can Eat: How Hungry Is America?* New York: Seven Stories Press, 2008.

Feeding America. https://www.feedingamerica.org/.

Fisher, Andrew. *Big Hunger: The Unholy Alliance between Corporate America and Anti-Hunger Groups.* Cambridge, MA: MIT Press, 2018.

Food Bank News. https://foodbanknews.com/.

Gottlieb, Robert, and Anupama Joshi. *Food Justice.* Cambridge, MA: MIT Press, 2010.

Mandyck, John, and Eric Schultz. *Food Foolish: The Hidden Connection between Food Waste, Hunger and Climate Change.* Palm Beach Gardens, FL: Carrier Corporation, 2015.

CHAPTER 2

History of Food Assistance Programs

If you want to know where you're going, it's important to know where you've been. Likewise, if we want to end hunger, it's important to understand the history of food assistance in our country. The development of most government-run food assistance programs in the 1960s, the rise of income inequality in the 1970s, and cuts to federal programs in the 1980s led to a model of food banking that has persisted for over forty years. While charitable food programs have evolved over time, broader reforms are long overdue. Examining our nation's response to hunger in recent decades prepares us to take on new strategies we can implement in our communities today.

Let's be clear: hunger is a preventable problem. That Americans (and most people around the world) experience food insecurity is a matter of access and power, not a lack of food. In 2018, 37 million Americans were food insecure, including one out of every nine adults and one out of every seven kids. We live in the wealthiest country on the planet. We waste approximately 40 percent of our food. These numbers don't add up. We can do better.

History of Federal Food Assistance

Charged with providing for the well-being of its citizens, the federal government runs several food assistance programs that are the first line of defense against hunger. The Supplemental Nutrition Assistance Program (SNAP, formerly called food stamps) was piloted during the Great Recession in 1939 and then became a permanent program in 1964. Fun fact—did you know that the National School Lunch program was created in 1946 to ensure that young men were nourished and capable of fighting in world wars? It's true. The School Breakfast Program and Summer Food Service Program were created in the late 1960s, and the Special Supplemental Nutrition Program for Women, Infants, and Children (WIC Program) was created in the early 1970s to ensure that women and children have basic nutrition.

However, during the 1970s, political and economic shifts triggered the growing divide in wages and wealth and help explain why food insecurity remains such a persistent problem despite the availability of multiple federal food assistance programs.

These and several other programs are the nutritional safety net that helps ensure Americans have enough food. Much has been written about these programs, they are closely regulated, and they are routinely monitored to evaluate their effectiveness. I include several resources at the end of this chapter where you can find more information. Research from the 1970s showed that federal food assistance programs including food stamps, School Lunch, and WIC worked to reduce malnutrition and hunger.

However, during the 1970s, political and economic shifts triggered the growing divide in wages and wealth and help explain why food insecurity remains such a persistent problem despite the availability of multiple federal food assistance programs. According to the Center on Budget and Policy Priorities and the Pew Research Center, income inequality (the income gap between those at the top of the economic ladder and those in the middle and lower end of the ladder) increased sharply starting in the 1970s. Many factors contribute to the income divide, including tax policies that benefit the wealthy, globalization, and a stagnant minimum wage that has not kept pace with inflation. These events and policies are structural factors that have kept wages down for many working people that, in turn, help create food insecurity. And they also led to the development of food banks and our charitable response to hunger.

The United States has a solid foundation of federal food assistance programs because citizens believed their government had a responsibility to provide an adequate safety net for its people. Yet during the early 1980s, the Reagan administration made drastic cuts to federal food programs, especially food stamps. Many people who were no longer eligible for food stamps were struggling to make ends meet. Those policy changes increased the need for food and set the stage for a very different approach to treating hunger. It was a movement away from government programs toward a reliance on the nonprofit sector and especially faith-based organizations to provide basic human services. President George H. W. Bush popularized the notion of a "thousand points of light" to encourage people to volunteer in their local communities.

In her book *Sweet Charity?*, Jan Poppendieck writes, "Perhaps emergency food has reassured the public that no one will starve, and thus given Congress and the president tacit permission, if not enthusiastic support, to dismantle the federal guarantee of minimum support for those in need." She wrote this eloquent and compelling argument in 1998, and it still rings true today.

What contributes to food insecurity today? It's not surprising if you think about our basic economic landscape. In 2019 and the beginning of 2020 before COVID-19, unemployment was at a record low. But having a job, or two jobs, no longer guarantees security. When I was a teenager in the 1980s, I made $3.35 per hour working minimum wage at various part-time jobs. My first job was at Lee's Famous Chicken, a fast-food restaurant, and I can still smell the grease if I try hard enough. The federal minimum wage increased to $7.25 per hour in 2009 but has remained the same for over ten years and clearly has not kept pace with inflation. The costs for virtually all goods and services have increased significantly since 2009, particularly the costs

"Perhaps emergency food has reassured the public that no one will starve, and thus given Congress and the president tacit permission, if not enthusiastic support, to dismantle the federal guarantee of minimum support for those in need."

for housing, child care, and health care. The idea of a "minimum" wage implies the minimum amount required to be able to afford the basic costs of living without relying on others for assistance. Clearly, this government protection is not being upheld.

In addition to providing low wages, many companies that hire minimum wage workers routinely hire people to work part-time to avoid paying for health insurance and other benefits. This means that many people are working one or two jobs but do not have health insurance, paid vacation days, or sick days. A single mom may decide to leave her kids at home because she can't afford child care and she can't afford to miss work.

And yet, in order to be eligible for government assistance, you cannot have any measurable savings or assets and need to show proof of poverty. There is often no incentive to save or build assets if you are receiving public assistance. When a family is working and starts to earn more than the limit for government assistance, they can experience what is often called the "cliff effect" because they are no longer eligible for assistance for food, housing, and child care. It can literally feel like falling off a cliff with no safety net. Families feel doomed to fail, with little hope of getting ahead. The very programs designed to help families can force tough decisions about work and create the need for, or dependence on, charitable food.

History of Food Banks

Today, a generation of young adults has never known a time without food pantries, food banks, and canned food drives. It wasn't always this way. The very first food bank, St. Mary's, opened in Phoenix, Arizona in 1967, founded by pioneer John van Hengel. By 1977, there were food banks in eighteen cities around the country. To unite these various food banks, America's Second Harvest (now Feeding America) was created as an umbrella association in 1979. It was in the 1980s, when hunger became an acute problem nationwide, that most food banks opened their doors. Today Feeding America is the largest antihunger organization, the nation's second largest charity, and a national network with two hundred food banks as members.

Over the past four decades, food banks have grown and expanded, typically funded with major capital campaigns, financed mainly by local donors, foundations, and corporations, to move into larger offices and warehouses in order to distribute more food. The warehouses serve as collection and distribution centers (think of large Costco stores). Food and other items are picked up or delivered to food banks by donors, including retail grocery store chains, food manufacturers, farmers, and other food distributors. The food is edible, but for various reasons is not marketed for sale or is past its prime. Companies are able to donate their goods and receive a tax break for their donations thanks to the Good Samaritan Hunger Relief Tax Incentive Act passed by Congress in 2000.

Food banks also order food from the federal government through The Emergency Food Assistance Program (TEFAP) and the Commodity Supplemental Food Program (CSFP). Other food collected during local food drives typically represents a mere 5 percent or less of the overall inventory found in food banks. Food bank staff and an army of volunteers help to sort and organize the food and then prepare it for distribution to local programs, such as food pantries, meal programs, community kitchens, after-school programs, and mobile programs.

While food banks started with a handful of staff members, they now have multiple departments, such as operations, programs, communications, human resources, development, and agency relations, and a board of directors. While food banks are nonprofits and are classified by the IRS as 501c(3) organizations, they have grown into multimillion-dollar enterprises. Food banks and food pantries can be found in nearly every community in America, and their growth and expansion since the 1980s show that these programs are not temporary or designed to treat a sudden disaster. Rather, food banks have become institutionalized in our society and are part of our community fabric.

While every food bank has its unique story, most share some common milestones. Many of these benchmarks have been shaped by leadership and funding opportunities from Feeding America to help build the capacity of food banks. The following is a very basic time line of the key phases and program development of food banks over the past few decades.

Rather, food banks have become institutionalized in our society and are part of our community fabric.

Food Banking Time Line and Milestones

Decade	Major milestones
1960s	First food bank created in 1967 in Phoenix, Arizona
1970s	Several early food banks created; Second Harvest (now Feeding America) established as a nationwide network of food banks
1980s	Food Banking 1.0: Majority of food banks created with limited staff and office space; moved to bigger space
1990s	Food Banking 2.0: Warehouse expanded; pounds of food increased
2000s	Food Banking 3.0: Additional programs added, such as mobile programs to distribute fresh produce and backpack programs; warehouse expanded again
2010s	Food Banking 4.0: Founding CEO retired; Supplemental Nutrition Assistance Program (SNAP) outreach undertaken; retail pickup programs established to collect perishable products from grocery stores; connections made between hunger and health; nutrition policies created; college pantries established; Closing the Hunger Gap conferences started; warehouse expansion continued
2020s	Food Banking 5.0: Pursue ending hunger strategies for long-term solutions; create community food hubs; collaborate with social justice and advocacy organizations; envision other strategies yet to come!

You can see that the trend has been for growth and expansion by food banks nationally. Indeed, food banks have traditionally measured their success by the number of pounds of food distributed each year. Food banks report their poundage to Feeding America and also to their boards of directors and in their annual reports to donors and supporters. Progress has largely focused on acquiring, sorting, and distributing more food, which requires larger warehouses, more cooler space, and more trucks to deliver the food. You can also see where we are headed and what is possible during our next decade.

Our national charitable food system has grown in scope and scale for over forty years; as a country, we have distributed billions of pounds of food to millions of Americans. Yet, the number of food insecure families remains high and the need has not gone away. That's because it takes more than food to end hunger. We have to move beyond food distribution if we're serious about solving this problem.

If we define hunger as a symptom of poverty caused by a broken system, and rooted in social inequalities, then the solution becomes quite different.

The Problem of Hunger, Redefined

If we define hunger as a lack of food, then the solution seems quite simple: grow, collect, and provide more food to those in need. This makes a lot of sense. In the simplest terms, aren't people hungry because they don't have enough food? This is largely how we as a society have defined and tackled hunger for the past forty years, by collecting and distributing more food to people who experience hunger. We've become very skilled at this. In 2018, we efficiently distributed 4 billion pounds of food. And this is a conservative estimate because it doesn't count the smaller programs and food banks that aren't affiliated with Feeding America. So we've tackled hunger with a lot of food. Except, the problem hasn't gone away.

If we define hunger as a symptom of poverty caused by a broken system, and rooted in social inequalities, then the solution becomes quite different. Tax laws and policies created in the 1970s have created dramatic income inequality. Lengthy applications and funding cuts limit participation in federal food programs. Systemic injustices based on race, ethnicity, and gender translate into communities of color that have higher rates of poverty and crime, more pollution and toxic water, lower-resourced schools, and fewer full-sized grocery stores. There are many reasons why people are food insecure, and these root causes include

- High cost of living, especially the cost of housing and lack of affordable housing;
- Stagnant wages that haven't kept pace with inflation;
- Limited employment opportunities and limited education and job training to access living wage jobs;
- Lack of access to affordable, healthy food, with fewer supermarkets in low-income areas;
- Loss of income due to divorce, job loss, or health problems;
- Disability issues, including mental and physical health problems and addictions;
- Higher rates of chronic diseases that cause high medical expenses, as well as lack of access to affordable health care;
- High cost and limited access to child care and other supportive resources for employment; and
- Systemic inequalities that make it difficult for some groups (especially those based on race, ethnicity, and gender) to get ahead.

Yes, addressing these other root causes is more complex, it's messy, it's politically charged, and it will be harder and take longer to solve. All true. But let's go back to the premise that providing billions of pounds of food to millions of Americans for almost forty years has not reduced the number of people who need food. In fact, rates of food insecurity closely mirror the federal poverty rate. In addition to distributing food today as a short-term safety net, if we really mean what we say, that we want to "end hunger," then we need to address these systemic causes to break the cycle of food insecurity. As one food bank staff member said recently, "You wouldn't put a Band-Aid on a gunshot wound." We are doing very good work to distribute food in our communities, but it is a short-term Band-Aid to a much larger problem.

From this broad perspective, in order to end hunger, we as a society need to advocate for policy changes such as a higher minimum wage and affordable health care that will alleviate poverty and inequity. At the organizational level, food banks can raise their collective voices to broaden advocacy efforts beyond SNAP to other antipoverty programs. Food banks and food pantries can do a better job of helping individuals address the root causes of hunger (by providing wraparound services and more than just food). Rather than working alone in silos, various community organizations can collaborate to provide services (including food) to build collective impact.

At the interpersonal level, the ways in which a food pantry is designed and operated can dramatically affect the experience of those who visit the program, either positively or negatively. Charitable food programs can work directly with individuals to provide information, social support, education, and access to services to help with longer-term assistance so they won't need to keep coming to the food pantry.

In her seminal work, *Sweet Charity?*, Jan Poppendieck argues that the growth of the charitable food system takes the government off the hook from providing a more fundamental social safety net. I completely agree. But here's the thing. We in the charitable food system took ourselves off the hook too. We thought our programs were going to be short-term, so we waited for the government to invest in broader solutions. We thought it was the government's responsibility to provide adequate social services and robust food programs, so we got busy collecting and distributing food.

But there are systemic limitations with how charitable food organizations are currently run that hold us back from helping people become food secure and self-sufficient.

Charitable food systems are doing good work and we are helping people get food for today. But there are systemic limitations with how charitable food organizations are currently run that hold us back from helping people become food secure and self-sufficient. The tools in this book show how to address these limitations and provide strategies for longer-term solutions. What if our success is measured not simply by the pounds of food we distribute but by the reduction in people who need our services? Or the number of people who are connected to additional services? Or the number of people who make fewer trade-off decisions between paying for food, rent, or medicine? Or the number of people who have improved health outcomes based on the food and services they receive? How do we shift our attention from providing short-term food supplies to a more robust set of community services that offer more sustainable, long-term assistance? It's helpful to think about the different levels of impact, from the individual, to the organization, to the community, to broader policy changes.

New Models

Looking for ways to address hunger at its root causes, several progressive food banks and innovative food access organizations convened the Closing the Hunger Gap conference in September 2013, which was hosted by the Community Food Bank of Southern Arizona. Subsequent conferences have been held every two years, and the network has grown to include resource sharing and network building outside the conferences. The Closing the Hunger Gap network seeks to expand hunger relief efforts beyond food distribution toward strategies that promote social justice and long-term solutions.

Over the past several years, many funders, supporters, and staff have begun to question the standard model of charitable food and are looking for new approaches. I've heard from some food bank staff members who said their food bank revised their strategic plan around 2015 and added language about "ending hunger" or "shortening the line," in addition to their traditional work of distributing food for people today. But the words on the page didn't always translate into programming or action. They believed in this broader mission, but they didn't know how to do the work. So even though the plan sounded good and looked great in a brochure, it wasn't something upon which they could readily act.

In 2018, Feeding America created an Ending Hunger Community of Practice so member food banks could learn and share strategies beyond food distribution, such as job training, case management, and SNAP outreach. At a recent Feeding America conference, a food bank staff member from Texas said, "We're on a journey to end hunger, but we need a roadmap, and we don't have a dashboard. We may be driving different cars, but we want some standardization." Many food banks are looking for direction and want the ability to use evidence-based programs and share best practices so we don't re-create the wheel. We want to move away from simply measuring outputs of pounds and measure outcomes that show meaningful progress for the people we serve. This book provides a direction for where we want to go, with examples of best practices and tangible action steps to fill your dashboard.

In the following pages, we will explore various ways to improve the charitable food system at the individual, organizational, and policy levels. I'll advocate for consolidating food pantries and creating community food hubs that offer a more dignified experience for guests and provide opportunities for individuals to build skills that will contribute to an individual family's food security. These types of holistic food pantries can also help empower individuals to become advocates for larger community and policy changes.

One excellent community food hub that has informed my approach and can serve as a template for innovative food pantries is called Freshplace.

Freshplace

Starting in 2006, three nonprofit organizations joined together to create a different type of food pantry. Foodshare, the regional food bank of Greater Hartford, Connecticut (where I work now), the Chrysalis Center, a social service agency, and the Junior League of Hartford had the vision to create a holistic food pantry in Hartford, Connecticut. Freshplace is designed like a grocery store so clients (or members as they are called) shop for their food, but they also meet with a case manager about twice a month to identify areas in their lives that are holding them back and receive referrals to community services such as SNAP, utility assistance, and GED classes or job training. Given my background in conducting research on food insecurity, when I heard about the idea of Freshplace in 2009, I met with the team that was designing the program. I began partnering with them to help launch the program and to evaluate its impact.

In one of my first meetings with the agencies that were designing the program, I mentioned that if we could show that this holistic type of pantry worked to improve food security, then it could serve as a model for other communities around the country. I am proud to say that we conducted the first rigorous evaluation of a food pantry program at Freshplace. After several years of planning, Freshplace held a grand opening and ribbon cutting in June of 2010.

The Freshplace evaluation was designed as a randomized control trial, which is considered a gold standard for research. We recruited people from a few other traditional food pantries that were within walking distance to Freshplace. After collecting baseline survey information, we asked people to pick a ball from a bag. If they chose a blue ball, they became part of our control group, and we told them we would conduct the survey again in four months. If they chose a red ball, they became our intervention group, and we invited them to go to Freshplace. In this

way, we were comparing similar people and then measuring the differences between those who went to Freshplace versus those who continued to go to traditional food pantries.

We followed more than 220 people over eighteen months to evaluate the program, and we found very significant differences. Over
one year, Freshplace members were less than half as likely to experience very low food security, had increases in self-sufficiency scores of
four points on a scale from eleven to fifty-five (which shows improvements in factors such as employment, education, housing, and health
insurance), and ate more fruits and vegetables by one serving per day
compared with the control group. People who went to Freshplace also
had significant improvements in their self-efficacy—in other words,
their confidence in their ability to make life changes—and were going
to food pantries less often compared with the control group. Aside
from the quantitative data, we heard wonderful qualitative stories
from Freshplace members who described what a positive difference
the program had on their lives. This was exciting and encouraging.

Some early graduates from Freshplace shared their enthusiasm with us:

- "Everybody is talking about Freshplace, that it's helpful to the fam-
  ily. You can't just run in, you have to make an appointment. There is
  no quarreling like at the food truck. There is respect there."
- "Freshplace has been great. When I have an appointment at 12:30
  they are ready for me. I don't have to wait in line."
- "Not just food, they help you with doctors and other things."
- "You meet a lot of different people from different walks of life at
  Freshplace."
- "My goal was to eat healthier, so I went to Cooking Matters.
  Learned to eat more vegetables, was able to get more fruits and veg-
  etables that I wasn't able to afford before. I'm eating healthier now."
- "The customer service, really try to help, food, employment, housing."

They came for the food, they appreciated the food, but they left with much more.

You can hear from these quotes the importance of how the program was delivered, with respect, customer service, and providing amenities beyond food. At the end of the second year of programming, the staff at the Chrysalis Center held focus groups with members to ask about their experience and opinions about the new food pantry. Mind you, the three organizations spent years and countless meetings designing the new program, and spent a lot of time thinking about what food would be offered and how they would provide the food. One of the shocking realizations from the focus groups was how little the members talked about the food at all. They talked about how they were treated by Jon Mitchell, the rockstar case manager, and by volunteers, how they didn't have to wait in line, how they became friends with other members, and about the other programs and services that helped them. They came for the food, they appreciated the food, but they left with much more.

More Than Food

From 2013 to today, I have collaborated with Urban Alliance, a wonderful faith-based organization in Greater Hartford. We spent time identifying the core components of Freshplace that we believed were most important for others to replicate. For simplicity, we call these the three *C*'s of culture, choice, and connection. You'll see each is described in more detail in upcoming chapters. As the work expanded and we began scaling it in other food pantries, we named our approach the More Than Food framework; the goal is to build the capacity of food banks and food pantries to address the root causes of hunger. As the name implies, it is our core belief that it takes more than food to end hunger.

A recent graduate from the Kelly Center for Hunger Relief, which is offering More Than Food in El Paso, Texas, had this to say about the program. "When I started the program, my life was very difficult. Fresh Start helped me to prioritize and set goals for myself. It helped me by being positive and having a better outlook on life." She is now an active volunteer at the Kelly Center and continues to take Zumba, yoga, and nutrition classes at the pantry.

We continue to learn from other food pantries who are now providing More Than Food and offering a welcoming culture, healthy choice, and connection. In 2020, there are several food pantries in Greater Hartford offering More Than Food, along with food pantries in Rhode Island and El Paso, Texas, and there is interest from several other states. A few of these pantries call their programs Fresh Start, which is a great way to describe the philosophy of the program. We have evidence to show this type of holistic food pantry works. Chapters 4–7 will provide tools for how to incorporate these best practices in your community.

The End of Hunger

Can we really end hunger? Often people remind me that hunger has existed since the beginning of time; they argue that there has always been hunger and there will always be hunger. I believe this is partly true. We will probably always need basic food distribution and shelter beds for people in our communities. People struggling with severe mental health issues, those who are permanently disabled, and seniors living on fixed incomes need ongoing aid. But this is a very small fraction of society and is a small percentage of the almost 40 million Americans who are food insecure.

There are large segments of people who should not need to rely on assistance and who do not want to rely on charity. How do we help shorten the line so food banks and food pantries can be available for those who need chronic care and also provide very short-term assistance for others to get back on their feet? This was how the charitable food system was first envisioned in the late 1970s and early 1980s.

> *Defining the problem of hunger as something beyond food is a new way of thinking.*

The situation has changed, income inequality has widened and wages have not kept pace, but our response has remained largely the same. It is time to change the way we think about hunger, how we design our programs to address hunger, and how we approach people who struggle with hunger. Unfortunately, we've taken this model of "feeding the hungry" and let it morph into massive operations serving families by the millions. We've let the federal social safety net erode and haven't held government accountable to provide for minimal services to combat poverty. How did we let this slope become so slippery?

Defining the problem of hunger as something beyond food is a new way of thinking. It requires courage to buck the status quo. If you've decided to pick up this book, I believe you are looking for a new way of doing business, some new strategies for helping people beyond three days' worth of food, and new solutions to this preventable problem. Freshplace and the More Than Food initiative, and many other model programs around the country, provide examples of how to approach our work differently.

Often, when we think about alleviating hunger, we focus almost entirely on the individual and almost entirely on collecting and distributing food. Paying attention to other political and structural factors can help identify different areas for change, within food pantries, food banks, in our communities, and in our policies.

This is not an either/or scenario—either we focus on individuals or we focus on policy change. What we need is a yes/and perspective.

YES, we need to build relationships with individuals at the micro-level and provide resources to help them become more food secure, AND we need policy changes at the macro-level to make sure there are adequate services and programs to help individual households thrive. YES, we need approaches for working individually with families to help with their unique situations, AND we need policy changes and laws to make it easier for individuals to get ahead. For example, a food bank can help an individual enroll in SNAP and invite her to testify before the state legislature when SNAP funding is threatened.

Time to Evolve

It's important to really understand where we've been and how we got to where we are today with charitable food so that we can chart our future course. For those of you who have been in this movement for a while, this should sound familiar and will hopefully resonate with your experiences. For those of you who have only been involved in smaller roles, perhaps coordinating an annual food drive, this may help add some context to the work you've been doing and provide some new ideas. And for those of you who are new to the charitable food sector, I hope this book will pave the path for new solutions and provide tools so you can get involved now.

One thing I have learned is that when you've seen one food pantry, you've seen one food pantry, and I think this holds true for food banks as well. Although there are food banks and food pantries in communities around the country, they look, feel, and operate very differently and are not regulated like federal food assistance programs. This is important when we think about sharing best practices. It may be hard to appreciate a new way of operating a food pantry when you've been involved with only one food pantry. I encourage you to visit different food pantries in your community to see how they run. If you work at a food bank, visit other food banks. Talk with different directors and ask about their history, their mission statement, their various programs, and their vision for the future. Be curious and ask questions. If you are part of the Feeding America network, use HungerNet to post and respond to questions. Let's learn from one another.

Feeding America and regional food banks can reinforce best practices to make sure they are implemented by food pantries and meal programs. At the same time, we should encourage diversity and uniqueness of local communities. In many ways, we want each food pantry to look and feel different than others because a pantry should reflect the local community and the people who shop there. Ideally, some of the staff and volunteers should be from the same ethnic background and speak the same language as people coming to get food. And the food should reflect the cultural preferences of people selecting the food.

Nationally, many food banks have experienced staff turnover, with the long-time CEO retiring in the past ten years, and newer directors taking the helm. This can cause tension among experienced staff members who are used to the old way of doing things but also opens doors for new ideas and initiatives. This book is about both micro and macro changes that are needed within our national charitable food system. We need all of you, longtime food bankers, weekend volunteers, and new ambassadors to help reinvent this system.

Action Steps

- Learn about the history and mission of your local food bank or food pantry.
- Find out if your food bank or food pantry has a strategic plan. If so, read it and see how it aligns with the topics in this book. If not, suggest that they create a plan to incorporate some of these strategies.

- Examine how much of your work is focused on food distribution for today versus helping to shorten the line and building long-term food security.
- Ask whether your programs are ready to offer more than food with additional services, workshops, coaching, or classes.
- Get ready to make a change. If not now, when?

Resources

Closing the Hunger Gap. https://www.thehungergap.org/.

Food Research and Action Center. https://www.frac.org.

Martin, Katie, Angela Colantonio, Katie Boyle, and Katherine Picho. "Self-Efficacy Is Associated with Increased Food Security in Novel Food Pantry Program." *Social Science & Medicine–Pop Health* (2016): 62–67. https://doi.org/10.1016/j.ssmph.2016.01.005.

Martin, Katie, Rong Wu, Michele Wolff, Angela Colantonio, and James Grady. "A Novel Food Pantry Program: Food Security, Self-Sufficiency, and Diet-Quality Outcomes." *American Journal of Preventive Medicine* 45, no. 5 (2013): 569–575. https://doi.org/10.1016/j.amepre.2013.06.012.

Poppendieck, Janet. *Sweet Charity? Emergency Food and the End of Entitlement.* New York: Viking Press, 1998.

Share Our Strength. https://www.shareourstrength.org/.

CHAPTER 3
A Paradigm Shift in How We Talk about Hunger

This book is about a paradigm shift to change the way we provide charitable food. It is about changing the conversation about hunger. To get to the root of the problem, we have to move the discussion beyond bread, pounds of food, and charity, to nutritious food, stability, and strength-based solutions. In this chapter, I describe terms used throughout the book and my rationale for using those specific terms. Words have power and they influence how we think about an issue and how we respond. So let's use our words wisely.

A Forty-Year Emergency?

Recent national research from Feeding America shows that most people who visit food pantries do so several times throughout the year, "reflecting persistent need," and many individuals are turning to food pantries as a regular source of food. According to a study conducted in 2014 for Feeding America, 63 percent of US households that go to charitable food programs plan for food from these programs as a part of their monthly household budget. This is not an unexpected situation but rather a routine strategy to make ends meet throughout the year.

Yet the term *emergency* is still used frequently by food banks, food pantries, and academics to describe our work, such as the emergency food system, emergency programs, and the emergency response to hunger. When the "emergency" has lasted more than forty years, I find this term to be inappropriate. It begs the question—where is the emergency?

> *When the "emergency" has lasted more than forty years, I find this term to be inappropriate. It begs the question— where is the emergency?*

The definition of emergency is "a serious, unexpected, and often dangerous situation requiring immediate action." This language matters because it helps shape our response to the problem and informs how we design our programs. When faced with an emergency, we need to focus on efficiency, trying to serve the most food to the most people in the least amount of time. Hurricanes and tornadoes are examples of how, in true emergencies, we need to supply food, bottled water, and blankets for people as quickly as possible. Both the situation and response are meant to be short-lived. We don't expect to treat hurricane victims for years, let alone decades.

How does this language translate into the mindset and mission of our food bank and food pantry programs? If our programs are designed as an emergency response, our services will be designed as short-term: we won't focus on the nutritional quality of food, we won't spend time getting to know the people seeking help, we won't evaluate our programs, and little thought will be given to long-term planning. The emphasis will be on keeping our heads down, doing the work, and trying just to serve the people in front of us.

During the COVID-19 pandemic of 2020, the charitable food system was thrown quickly into emergency response mode. The early weeks were focused on disaster relief and adjusting systems to respond to social distancing and health concerns. The pandemic is a reminder of what a true emergency feels like. But even though the health crisis is an emergency, the way we respond can be strategic and reflect our core values. Hopefully by the time you are reading this book we are on the other side of the pandemic and incorporating best practices for dealing with the chronic nature of food insecurity.

Does your food bank or food pantry have a mission statement? Do the words reflect your current programming and the direction you want for your organization, or could they be updated? Does your food bank or food pantry use "emergency" language in your website or communications?

The landscape of food banking has changed, and so must our language. Let's shift our view from treating hunger as an emergency and focus more on prevention and planning. Otherwise, we will continue to provide short-term Band-Aids for another forty years. One way to think about this is a paradigm shift from "emergency to empowerment." Think about the power of those words. Moving our programming away from emergency services allows us to address the underlying root causes of hunger and to help empower people to become stable and self-sufficient. And if and when a true emergency hits, like it did with COVID-19, food pantries and food banks can help support the delivery of short-term supplies of food and then return to their more fundamental work of long-term solutions.

Food Bank versus Food Pantry

Even though there are regional food banks serving basically every geographic region in the United States, and there are food pantries in nearly every community in our country, it is amazing how many people do not know the difference between the two, or use the terms interchangeably. A food bank serves a geographic region, often several counties and sometimes a whole state. Food banks have a large warehouse for collecting and storing food donations that are then distributed to smaller food programs such as food pantries and meal programs or shelters. A food pantry provides food directly to individuals in the community. I enjoy seeing the amazement of many visitors when they walk through our food bank for the first time because you can tell they were envisioning a much smaller operation, perhaps in the basement of a church.

Understanding the difference between a food bank and a food pantry is important because they serve very different roles in a community, and we want to be clear about with whom we are working. When someone says they went to a food bank, but they really mean a food pantry, it's confusing. If someone has never visited a food bank and has only seen a food pantry, they may not appreciate the scale and impact of the work done by a regional food bank. This misnaming gets tricky because some small food pantries call themselves a food bank. Some food banks, like Foodshare, do not have food bank in their names. Some regions use different terms. For example, in Minnesota and Vermont, food pantries are typically called food shelves, but they may reference that they are called food pantries in other parts of the country. What we call food pantries in the United States are called food banks in Canada. I know, this is confusing! But for this book, we're focused on the charitable food system in the United States.

Understanding the difference between a food bank and a food pantry is important because they serve very different roles in a community, and we want to be clear about with whom we are working.

It is important to use the correct terms when we're describing food banks and food pantries, if for no other reason than to clarify and standardize our work. New organizations such as colleges, hospitals, and clinics are beginning to partner with food banks and food pantries, and we would be wise to make sure everyone has a clear understanding of these terms and uses them appropriately. The clearest way to see the difference between a food bank and a food pantry is to go visit one. Please, go visit your local food bank and visit at least one local food pantry. You'll see the difference. Then, hopefully, we can stop confusing the two and describing them as the same thing.

Defining the Terms *Food Insecurity* and *Hunger*

Up until the 1980s in the United States, we simply talked about the problem of hunger. In the mid- to late 1980s, questions arose about the severity of the problem because we didn't have a standard definition of hunger in the United States, and we didn't have solid estimates of how many people were actually hungry. Conservative legislators justified cuts to federal food assistance programs, arguing that we didn't really know how many people needed food. We have all felt the physical sensation of hunger before mealtimes, but we were clearly talking about a different situation, and we needed a better way to define and quantify the problem.

Researchers began to study the issue of hunger and also developed a standard definition of food insecurity that better described the broader spectrum of hunger in the context of a wealthy country such as the United States. The nonprofit Life Sciences Research Office convened an expert panel to define food security in 1989. According to the definition, food security means access to enough food for an active, healthy life. To be food secure, you need at a minimum (1) the availability of nutritionally adequate and safe foods, and (2) the ability to acquire acceptable foods in socially acceptable ways (without having to use emergency food programs, scavenging, stealing, or employing other coping strategies).

Think about that. By this definition, you would be considered food insecure if you do not have access to nutritious food, not just a sufficient amount of food. It would still take many years before we became serious about nutritional standards for our food assistance programs. You would also be considered food insecure if you have to use a food pantry or community kitchen as a coping strategy to get food. In 1989, the very act of having to rely on charitable food programs was described as socially unacceptable, similar to stealing or taking food out of a trash can. No wonder there is stigma and embarrassment around going to a food pantry. We don't talk about federal food programs in this way. Having your child receive a reduced-priced school lunch or applying for WIC isn't considered a socially unacceptable coping strategy.

The definition for food security is still used today, but we don't stress the additional requirements of not using emergency food programs as a coping strategy. Otherwise, our estimates of how many people are food insecure would be even higher than they are.

Food insecurity is a much more accurate term for describing the experience of millions of Americans who worry about having enough food at the end of the week or the end of the month. But food insecurity doesn't carry the same emotional weight or simplicity as the term hunger. It is more compelling to describe a child going to bed hungry or families that don't know where their next meal is coming from. But these phrases can distort the problem when they're not backed up with facts.

Measurement of Food Insecurity and Hunger

During the 1980s, pioneering researchers conducted surveys to find an accurate way to measure hunger and food insecurity. They asked low-income families about their coping strategies when they did not have enough money for food. Kathy Radimer and colleagues from Cornell University and the Community Childhood Hunger Identification

Project sponsored by the nonprofit Food Research and Action Center made the early attempts to measure the severity and scope of the problem of hunger in the United States.

Starting in 1995, the US Census Bureau included these eighteen questions in their annual Current Population Survey, and we have years of national estimates for the number and characteristics of people who experience food insecurity.

These researchers held hundreds of conversations with low-income families and found that they used similar strategies when they were running out of money. Adults first worried about having enough food, then they cut back on the quality and variety of their own food, and, as a last resort, they cut back on their kids' food. Parents tend to shield their kids from food insecurity as much as possible, so adults will cut back on the size of their meals or skip meals and in the most severe cases will reduce the quantity of their kids' meals. This research led to the development of the eighteen-item standardized questionnaire to measure food insecurity, which has been validated in many different populations, languages, and settings. Starting in 1995, the US Census Bureau included these eighteen questions in their annual Current Population Survey, and we have years of national estimates for the number and characteristics of people who experience food insecurity.

The eighteen questions are scored to classify households into four levels: high, marginal, low, and very low food security. The questions are asked about a household's experiences over the last twelve months. To be considered marginally food secure, a household may answer yes to worrying about having enough food because they were running out of money to buy more, but they have no reductions in the quality or quantity of their food. When households answer yes to not just worrying about enough food but cutting back on the quality and variety of their food, then they are classified as food insecure. At the most extreme, when a household experiences "very low food security" it means the adults are skipping meals or cutting back on the size of their children's meals or not eating for a whole day because they do not have enough money to buy more. The people in this category are experiencing hunger, not just food insecurity. I can tell you that in my many years of asking these eighteen questions, while it is rare, I have had families respond yes to all eighteen questions. I've included the website with information on the US Department of Agriculture (USDA) food security measure at the end of the chapter.

The USDA reports national estimates for each of the four levels of food insecurity and describes characteristics of people who are most likely to be in each category. The most recent estimates show that 11 percent of US households (14.3 million) were food insecure at some time during 2018, including 4 percent (5.6 million households) who had very low food security. These rates have been relatively steady over time, with a low of 10 percent food insecurity in 1999, 11 percent in 2002 and 2007, and a big spike during the Great Recession in 2008, reaching a high of 15 percent in 2011. We will likely see another spike during 2020 in response to COVID-19.

This may be more detail about the food security screener than you care to know. But a lot of research and science has gone into these measurements to provide accurate descriptions and statistics on the people who are food insecure in our country. We have reliable, nationally representative data on food insecurity dating back to 1995. We have effective tools to measure and quantify the otherwise abstract concept of "hunger." There is also

We have effective tools to measure and quantify the otherwise abstract concept of "hunger."

a shorter six-item questionnaire to measure food insecurity, and even a two-item questionnaire that is recommended to be used in clinical settings like hospitals and health clinics, particularly those serving kids.

For those of us who are involved in charitable food assistance, it is important to understand these measures and these different terms. For academics who are interested in conducting research in food pantries, it is helpful to use the standardized measures. Check out the resources at the end of this chapter for more information about the definitions and survey questions. By using the standard tools, we will use common terms and can compare data from local programs to national estimates.

So then, here is our challenge. On the one hand, we want to use accurate language based on years of solid research to define and quantify who is food insecure. On the other hand, it is much more evocative and conversational to talk about hunger and to claim that millions of Americans go to bed hungry each night. How do we use accurate information without being too technical and confusing for our supporters? How do we paint a clear picture while trying to compel donors to send money to support our work? How can we use simple and compelling language that is also supported by research?

When I describe food insecurity, I typically describe how millions of people have to worry about getting enough food at the end of the week or the end of the month (not their next meal or tonight). These descriptions come directly from the questions used to measure food insecurity. I describe how many people have to make tough decisions between paying for food or paying for rent or medicine. And even though I prefer the more accurate term food insecurity, you'll see that throughout the book I'll refer to hunger too. We don't want to get too caught up in the trees that we can't see the forest.

Fundraising Appeals

Some of you may remember the TV commercials with Sally Struthers pleading with people to send money immediately or else a starving African child might die of malnutrition right in her arms. Unfortunately, many antihunger organizations still use this strategy of guilting people into sending money and painting a sad, terrible image of hunger. It's time to evolve to describe not just the needs of the people we serve but also their hopes and strengths.

Think about your fundraising appeals and the way you describe your work to existing and potential donors. Do you pull on heartstrings by describing a family's plight and struggle with having no food in their refrigerator? I believe many of our donors are tired of receiving these appeals. Instead, can you describe a positive example of how a family got back on their feet after receiving your services? Can you tell a story of a client who no longer needs to go to the pantry and now volunteers? You can use ethical storytelling by listening to the experiences of the people you serve and asking their permission to share their stories. Staff at Foodshare recently interviewed a woman who used a pantry in our network. After the interview, the woman thanked the staff for listening to her story. She said she felt like a weight was off her shoulders because she was able to share her experience, which might help others. Many people want to share their story and feel heard. Many donors want to know that their money is going to improve a family's situation rather than to treat a never-ending problem.

Many donors want to know that their money is going to improve a family's situation rather than to treat a never-ending problem.

When we target our fundraising efforts by saying that the need is always getting bigger and the problem is always getting worse, we provide an inaccurate picture and do a disservice to our supporters. When food insecurity rates decrease, typically during healthy economic times, we in the antihunger sector should see this as good news and an indicator that people are more likely to have enough food.

We should use the data to understand what social, economic, and political drivers have contributed to the reduction in food insecurity. Did a state pass a higher minimum wage law? Did unemployment rates decrease? Who has not benefited from the strong economy? Who is food insecure despite working one or two jobs? Being knowledgeable about these trends and telling this story is important too. Similarly, if we only describe the problem of hunger in terms of pounds of food and lack of food, we take our eyes off the more fundamental root causes of food insecurity.

Scarcity Mentality: How to Move from Deficit-Based to Strength-Based Language

A key issue that is holding us back from really tackling and ending hunger is the focus on not having enough. Within charitable food work, and in other nonprofit sectors too, we describe this concept as the scarcity mentality. This mindset affects both people living in poverty and people working in food banks and food pantries. Scarcity mentality is the concern that there isn't enough—food, money, support, time, resources. And when you're worried that there isn't enough, you make tough choices and create various coping mechanisms. You don't try new opportunities. You lose hope. You stay in your comfort zone.

When you're struggling with food insecurity, you cut back on the size of your meals, buy less expensive food, send your kids to a neighbor's house to eat a meal, buy more food at the beginning of the month when food stamps replenish, and skip meals when money is low. You make difficult trade-offs between paying for food, medicine, utilities, or rent, often on a monthly basis. When you do not have enough money, you focus on lack. You don't have the luxury to plan or save when you are focused on today. These coping strategies are often necessary in order to survive and get by.

Dr. Sendhil Mullainathan and colleagues at the University of Chicago have conducted several studies on scarcity. They describe how living in poverty and having a scarcity mindset forces individuals to focus on short-term needs and what is lacking rather than on other priorities. Dealing with scarcity can impact one's cognitive function and sense of self-control. Their research shows how scarcity can explain behaviors such as overborrowing. Using a payday lender or check cashing service with a ridiculously high interest rate seems like an obvious mistake. But when you need money immediately, especially if you don't have a traditional banking account, this choice seems to make perfect sense. When you focus attention on what you don't have, it leads you to make decisions that provide short-term gain but will hinder long-term well-being and, in the long term, will only make matters worse.

The program Bridges Out of Poverty calls this the tyranny of the moment—when you are focused on survival mode—paying enough rent to not get evicted or enough money to keep the lights on, taking two buses and two hours to go to a store because you can save $0.29 on canned beans. These decisions keep people from future planning and thriving. Recognizing this mentality is important and can inform how we design our programs and services. We can increase empathy and build in flexibility to our programs to accommodate the chaotic and often unstable situations of the people we serve. We can focus on ways not just to provide food but to build more stability so people can focus on bigger goals.

Another example is the language we use to describe our programs. A financial literacy class may be well intentioned but may not seem relevant for people with a scarcity mindset. I spoke with a food pantry guest a few years ago who talked about his reason for not joining a budget coaching class. He said, "I don't have two pennies to scratch together. What am I going to budget?" The class may be better received and attended if we describe it by simply saying, "Do you want to save more money this month?" A great way to find a name for a new program is to ask people who are likely to use the program for their opinions. Describe what the program will involve and what the potential benefits will be. How do they describe it, and what would encourage them to participate? Use their words to describe the program.

Scarcity Mentality in Organizations

It is not surprising to hear a scarcity mentality at the individual level, and this has been documented routinely by Feeding America and the USDA Economic Research Service food security reports. But we often hear a scarcity mentality at the organizational level, too, and among food pantry directors who are focused on lack. This mindset is often present in the way that directors and volunteers operate food pantries. We don't have enough—fill in the blanks—space, food, volunteers, equipment, money, time. And therefore, we just need to get by and provide basic needs. We can't plan or think about the future because we are worried about today.

Nearly every food pantry I have visited sets limits on how often people can visit the pantry or how much food they can take or sets up systems for volunteers to shop with clients to make sure the clients don't take too much food. I understand that pantries do not have unlimited resources, but it may be time to reevaluate these policies to make sure the strict limits for clients are justified.

Aside from the way a food pantry distributes food, the scarcity mentality manifests in more fundamental ways too. It can lead to a deficit-based view of the pantry, and worse yet, it can extend into seeing the deficits in others. Viewing clients as having many needs and problems can lead to a feeling that they are lazy or not very smart or cannot be trusted. The words and tone used when people come to a pantry can reinforce a scarcity mentality, and the language posted on signs can discourage clients. When people arrive, are they told sternly to stay in line? Do signs remind clients that they can take only two cans of soup? Can you get the same message across by using more welcoming signs and language?

The scarcity mentality can also create competition between nonprofit organizations, including food banks, food pantries, and other social service providers. If you believe that resources are scarce, and you are applying for grant funding, you are less likely to collaborate or share ideas with other groups because you worry that they will steal your ideas and they will get the grant instead of your organization. I believe we will all be better stewards of grant funding when we collaborate and partner with others. In fact, many funders now require or strongly suggest some type of collaboration between organizations to avoid silos where organizations work alone.

It is hard to build capacity within a food bank or a food pantry that is stuck in a scarcity mentality. When volunteers or staff are focused on not having enough, they can be reluctant to try something new. Because there are a lot of people with immediate needs for food, it is easy to get stuck in treating the emergency and providing Band-Aids rather than addressing the chronic problem of food insecurity with a more holistic approach. It's safer to stay in the status quo and simply hand out food.

But we have to be careful because our beliefs become our thoughts, our thoughts become our words, our words become our actions, our actions become our habits, and our habits become our values.

A Focus on Strengths

The opposite of scarcity mentality is a strength-based approach and a feeling of abundance. The term *strength-based* can be used to describe both a way of seeing others and how services are delivered: recognizing the inherent strengths in others, providing services without judgment, believing there is enough food for everyone, trusting that if you allow clients to choose their food they will take what they need but not more. Many organizations conduct needs assessments to identify weaknesses in a community. Some organizations are starting to conduct asset mapping to identify the various resources and opportunities within a community. When we see people in a food pantry line as having strengths, dreams, and goals, we can leverage their contributions.

Now it very well may be true that you are dealing with a lack of volunteers or space or food. But if you commit to trying a new approach, it can help you get creative and think outside the box. This is how innovation and reinvention take place. If you need more volunteers, can you talk with guests at your pantry and ask if some would like to volunteer to help out? Talk with other social service agencies that utilize volunteers and see how you might collaborate. If you want to expand your services, look for new funders who haven't funded your basic needs program but might fund your health promotion class or budgeting workshop. Think about other available space that could be converted for new programs, or think about how you might reconfigure your existing space for different uses. Think about how you might collaborate with another agency to refer some of your clients to programs offered by that local agency.

When we see people in a food pantry line as having strengths, dreams, and goals, we can leverage their contributions.

Imagine if we take a strength-based approach when providing charitable food and running food programs. We would recognize that everyone has strengths that they bring to the table, even though they are going through tough times. They have something to share and offer. We would see possibilities and opportunities for growth, both for the people we serve and for our organizations.

In this book, you'll notice that I often use the term *guest* to refer to people who visit food pantries. This is intentional. Typically we use the term *client*, but by referring to the people we serve as guests, we can center our charitable food work on customer service and hospitality and create a better overall experience.

Strength-based Programs

One of the food pantries that is using our More Than Food framework is a model food pantry in El Paso, Texas, that I mentioned at the start of the book. They recently changed their name from the Kelly Memorial Food Pantry to the Kelly Center for Hunger Relief to better describe their mission. They have a large banner inside the pantry that says, "Welcome to Your Fresh Start." They converted their traditional food pantry to a client choice pantry where guests select their own food. Some graduates of their program now come to the pantry to volunteer. This is essential. Graduates can provide great word of mouth to recruit new clients and to reduce stigma about coming to the pantry for assistance. The Kelly Center partners with other social service agencies to enroll clients in local programs. Clearly, they have made a shift from emergency to empowerment.

Several food banks offer job training programs because they recognize that clients want to build skills and need more than just food. We have trained coaches to work individually with food pantry clients to set goals toward stability and health. The coaches describe how their clients have successfully completed GED programs, enrolled in community college, gained cooking skills, are eating more fruits and vegetables, are managing their diabetes, and are pursuing other goals. The coaches are trained in motivational interviewing skills, which is a strength-based approach used frequently in social work. The coaches see the best in their clients and help empower them to set and reach goals. I describe these in more detail in chapter 7, but if we want to help people achieve these types of goals, we first need to recognize that they have strengths in addition to needs.

Suggested New Language

To help you consider the language that you use, the chart below provides some examples of old-school language that I believe is outdated and then suggests new language that is strength-based, is more accurate, or uses an equity lens to be more inclusive. I also provide a brief rationale to describe the differences between the two descriptions. I hope this will give you some ideas for the words you choose for your work.

Suggested Language

Old school	Suggested language	Rationale
Feeding hungry people Feeding the hungry	Ensure everyone has access to enough food Provide food for people who are food insecure	We aren't actually feeding others, nor do we want to. This is a paternalistic and degrading approach. We feed our pets. People can feed themselves. Also, saying "the hungry" creates an "us versus them" mentality. Using people-first language puts a person before a diagnosis or a problem, describing what a person "has" rather than asserting what a person "is."
100,000 people are going to bed hungry tonight 100,000 people don't know where their next meal is coming from	100,000 people worry about having enough food for their families 100,000 people have to make difficult decisions between paying for food, rent, utilities, or medical bills	National statistics on food security are based on questions related to experiences over one year, so it is inaccurate to say that all those who are food insecure are going to bed hungry tonight. Food insecurity is more of a chronic problem than an immediate need for food for the next meal.

Emergency food programs	Food pantries, community kitchens, meal programs Community partners Partner programs	When we think of an emergency, we think of short-term responses. Food insecurity is more of a chronic problem rather than an emergency situation. "Emergency" food programs should be reserved for natural disasters or a health crisis.
Focus on pounds of food or even meals' worth of food	Reduction in food insecurity or increase in self-sufficiency Percent of clients who rated their visit to the food pantry as good or excellent Percentage of people who made fewer trade-off decisions between paying for food, rent, or medicine	The focus of providing more food to more people every year has not, and will not, solve the problem of hunger. We want to measure the impact of our work in terms of outcomes. While pounds are easy to calculate and quantify, they are not the solution to the problem. Showing growth in pounds can distract us from more holistic approaches.
Focus on total pounds rather than nutritional quality of those pounds	Describe overall pounds in terms of nutritional quality, such as green, yellow, and red to highlight healthy pounds of food Percentage of people who had improved health outcomes based on the food and services they received	As we promote health and nutrition, we also need to measure the nutritional quality of the pounds we distribute. Simply focusing on total pounds can mask the health consequences of the food we distribute. Containers of soda weigh more than green leafy vegetables but have a much different effect on the health of the people we serve.
Clients	Guest, customer, member, participant	When we view the people we serve as guests or customers at our programs, we place more emphasis on customer service and pay attention to the guest experience.

Action Steps

- Let's stop using the term *emergency* to describe our programs and approach to hunger.
- Know the difference between a food bank and a food pantry and use the terms appropriately. Help inform others about the difference between a food bank and food pantry.
- Take a critical look at the words you use on your website, in your fundraising appeals, in research articles, and in your programming. Switch from old-school language to newer language described in this chapter.
- Ask food pantry guests to list or describe one thing they are most proud of and post these responses on a bulletin board.
- Is your organization focused primarily on not having enough? Think about the area you feel is lacking most and collaborate with others to build resources and strength in this area.
- If you are designing a new program at your food bank or food pantry, think about the language you use to describe it. If possible, ask people who are your intended customers about their opinions for how to describe the program.
- Take one step, if not you, then who?

Resources

Community Food Centres Canada: Good Food Is Just the Beginning. https://cfccanada.ca/en/Home.

Mani, Anandi, Sendhil Mullainathan, Eldar Shafir, and Jiaying Zhao. "Poverty Impedes Cognitive Function." *Science* 341, no. 6149 (2013): 976–980. https://doi.org/10.1126/science.1238041.

Martin, Katie, Maryellen Shuckerow, Christine O'Rourke, and Allison Schmitz. "Changing the Conversation about Hunger: The Process of Developing

Freshplace." *Progress in Community Health Partnerships* 6, no. 4 (2012): 429–434. https://doi.org/10.1353/cpr.2012.0056.

US Department of Agriculture. "Definitions of Food Security." https://www.ers.usda.gov/topics/food-nutrition-assistance/food-security-in-the-us/definitions-of-food-security/.

US Department of Agriculture. "Food Security in the U.S." https://www.ers.usda.gov/topics/food-nutrition-assistance/food-security-in-the-us/.

CHAPTER 4
A Welcoming Culture

Take a minute to think about a food pantry with which you are familiar. How does it feel when you walk into the pantry? How are people greeted and treated? Do people stand outside in the rain, snow, or heat waiting to get food? Do volunteers warn clients to stay in line and wait their turn? Is the atmosphere in the line stressful, where tensions run high and arguments can erupt over people cutting the line or getting more food than others? What does the pantry look like inside? Is there a waiting area with chairs? Is it well lit and organized or is this the last place you'd want your neighbor to see you go?

The emphasis of many pantries is on efficiency. The focus is on finding the quickest and easiest way to get food to the most people who need it. However, efficiency is not always the same as effectiveness, and it can detract from equity. What we may gain in speed can be lost in the quality of service. Small indignities can add up to make the experience of visiting the pantry humiliating. When people take the step to go to a food pantry to receive charitable food, we want to avoid injuring their self-esteem and self-respect.

There is already a lot of negative stigma attached to going to a food pantry. This stigma is the reason why many people choose not to visit food pantries even when they do not have enough to eat. It may also contribute to the higher rates of depression among people experiencing food insecurity compared with those who are food secure. Visiting a food pantry is often humbling and embarrassing. It doesn't have to be this way.

Visiting a food pantry is often humbling and embarrassing. It doesn't have to be this way.

Unfortunately, I have witnessed stigmatizing food pantries that are run by well-meaning volunteers who, I believe, are doing their best to meet the need in their communities. To be clear, we don't create stigma on purpose. Staff and volunteers at food pantries have good intentions. However, too often traditional food pantries are set up with people waiting in long lines, and when they reach the front of the line they are handed a bag of food. Or clients wait while volunteers select and bag the food for them. The implicit, or sometimes verbalized, message is that clients should be grateful for what they get. The function of the pantry is to provide food and not much else. It is a transaction. We can do better. As you can see from many examples throughout the book, many food pantries are evolving. We can create food pantries that are welcoming, dignified, and empowering. You can think of this as the culture of a food pantry.

One goal of this book is to highlight ways to move our food pantry operations from transactional, to relational, and ultimately to transformational. To move in this direction, it is important to recognize that people who are living in poverty and who are food insecure may have experienced trauma and are more likely to struggle with depression and anxiety. Being poor is isolating and stressful; it can be hard to seek help at a food pantry.

> *The ways in which our food pantries are designed and operated can either add stress, anxiety, and stigma or they can uplift, encourage, and empower.*

The ways in which our food pantries are designed and operated can either add stress, anxiety, and stigma or they can uplift, encourage, and empower. In this chapter I highlight multiple ways that any food pantry, regardless of budget or size, can create a more welcoming environment. But first, let's understand why this is so important.

Food Insecurity, Stress, and Isolation

Over the past ten years, more attention has focused on the connection between hunger and health and the fact that food insecurity is associated with chronic diseases. Yet this attention is still largely focused on physical health, such as high blood pressure and type 2 diabetes. That food insecurity is also associated with mental health complications such as anxiety and depression, and the mental toll of worrying about having enough food for one's family, have not garnered as much attention.

One of my colleagues, Dr. Hilary Seligman, a professor at the University of California–San Francisco, has done extensive research on food insecurity and health outcomes, particularly type 2 diabetes. She created a conceptual framework to highlight the cycle of food insecurity and increased risk for chronic diseases. For example, when you are food insecure, you use coping strategies such as eating less nutritious food because it costs less, which can lead to chronic disease. When you have a chronic disease, your health-care expenses go up and you can have a hard time keeping a job, which decreases your income. With reduced income, you have to make difficult decisions between paying for food and paying other bills, which will lead to food insecurity. One of the things I like most about Hilary's framework is that she highlights how stressful it is to deal with these coping strategies and trade-off decisions.

It is stressful to be food insecure. In fact, the standard USDA questionnaire used to determine if a household is food insecure begins by asking if the following statement is true: "We worried whether our food would run out before we had money to buy more." The worry of not having enough food at the end of the week or the end of the month is the crux of experiencing food insecurity. Research shows that people experiencing food insecurity have increased risk for depression and anxiety. This may help explain why customers often line up hours before a food pantry will open because they worry there won't be enough food for everyone. The fear created by living with poverty and food insecurity is, in fact, a type of trauma.

Food Insecurity and Trauma

Over the past few years, social service providers and researchers have raised the importance of trauma-informed care, but this is still a very new topic for food banks and food pantries. According to the American Psychiatric Association, a traumatic experience involves a threat to one's physical or emotional well-being and elicits intense feelings of helplessness, terror, and lack of control. A traumatic experience can change a person's view of themselves, their surroundings, and the people around them. Research

Trauma can be both a cause and an effect of food insecurity.

shows that potentially traumatic events in childhood can have negative, lasting effects on health and well-being. The Adverse Childhood Experiences Study, conducted by the Centers for Disease Control and Prevention and Kaiser Permanente, highlights how poverty reinforces trauma and difficult experiences.

Experiencing some type of trauma, whether it is physical, sexual, or emotional, can make it hard to finish school or keep a job, which leads to less financial stability and less food security. In turn, not having enough food is traumatic. You'll notice this is a chicken and egg scenario. It's a vicious cycle. Trauma can be both a cause and an effect of food insecurity.

Trauma involves a painful or distressing experience that often results in lasting mental and physical effects. Here are some things to consider. If you are struggling with poverty and food insecurity, you are also more likely to

- Attend funerals and know people who die prematurely;
- Live in a neighborhood or an apartment that has environmental toxins and pests;
- Have unreliable transportation or child care, which can make it difficult to keep appointments and maintain a job;
- Have suffered domestic violence and decided to leave a violent relationship;
- Live in a zip code with a higher crime rate and lower life expectancy than other, food secure neighborhoods;
- Have suffered physical or emotional abuse; or
- Make difficult trade-off decisions on a monthly basis between paying for rent, food, utilities, or medicine.

The worry, anxiety, stress, and depression that coexist with food insecurity can hinder stability and a person's ability to thrive. People who are food insecure are often living with chaos and crisis. According to the Trauma-Informed Organizational Toolkit (listed in the resources at the end of this chapter), understanding traumatic stress and how it impacts people is critical for human service programs. This includes those of us who are involved with charitable food programs.

The worry, anxiety, stress, and depression that coexist with food insecurity can hinder stability and a person's ability to thrive.

Coping Strategies

By understanding the impact of trauma and the traumatic nature of food insecurity, we can better empathize with the people we serve. We can recognize that many behaviors that may seem ineffective or unhealthy today are in fact adaptive responses to past traumatic experiences. According to the Toolkit, "Trauma impacts how people access services. People who have experienced on-going trauma may view the world and other people as unsafe. Those who have repeatedly been hurt by others may come to believe that people cannot be trusted. This lack of trust makes it difficult for families to ask for help, trust providers, or form relationships."

If you spend time at food pantries or meal programs, these coping behaviors will likely be familiar. People may argue and get agitated if someone appears to be cutting in line. People may become upset if volunteers seem to be giving more food to others or taking more food for themselves. People will line up hours before a pantry is scheduled to open, even if directors make it clear that no food will be disbursed before the set time. The sheer nature of waiting a long time in line will heighten anxiety and stress. This too is a vicious cycle. When you are worried about having enough food, these coping strategies may help you make sense of your uncertain situation. It's part of the scarcity mindset. Seemingly irrational behavior (yelling at a volunteer about one loaf of bread) starts to make sense when we understand that it stems from past traumas and stress.

Recognizing that food insecurity is traumatic will help us move from transactions to customer service. Rather than simply providing food to people as quickly as possible, we will take the time to acknowledge our guests and build relationships with them. To begin this transition, let's consider some ideas for creating a more welcoming, dignified, and empowering culture at food pantries and meal programs.

Human Interaction

When you visit a hotel or restaurant, the staff use your name when you check in, they use eye contact, smile, and make small talk. One way to provide a welcoming and dignified environment at a charitable food program is to refer to the people you serve as guests or customers who are choosing to visit your program. When we think about the people we serve as guests, our focus will shift from food distribution to hospitality, and we can think of creative ways to provide customer service. I've described how the tools in this book are like a menu from which you can chose to reinvent the way you run your food bank or food pantry. Creating a welcoming and empowering environment is like the special sauce you can use to add flavor. The key ingredient is providing good service.

Designate one of your regular volunteers to serve as a "greeter," whose main job is simply to welcome people to the pantry, offer a smile, and greet people by name. These volunteers should wear name badges and introduce themselves to new customers to build rapport. The greeter can set a tone that is relaxed and assures people that there will be enough food for everyone. Choose a person who is friendly and outgoing and who will not be overly strict or stern. This could also be one of your regular customers who has the time to volunteer and who may find pride in giving back to others in the community.

Empathy versus Sympathy

To help empower others requires empathy and connection. Empathy means feeling *with* someone else about their situation, struggles, and dreams. It is different from having sympathy *for* someone else, which can actually create a divide rather than a connection. Brené Brown's book *Dare to Lead* and Robert Lupton's book *Toxic Charity* both highlight the difference between doing for others, which can be alienating, versus doing with others, which builds connection and empathy. Consider the differences between the two:

- Sympathy—I'm so sorry for you. I don't understand your situation, but it looks pretty bad. It must be embarrassing. You probably don't want to talk about it.
- Empathy—I see you, I want to hear about your situation, and I want to know more. Many people have had a similar experience, you're not alone, and we want to help.

In *Toxic Charity*, Lupton says that "to effectively impact a life, a relationship must be forged, trust built, accountability established. And this does not happen in long, impersonal lines of strangers." So first, we need to create opportunities for staff, volunteers, and guests to interact and get to know one another. This can start with a greeter who makes eye contact, smiles, and says hello to individuals when they arrive at the pantry. Rather than having volunteers bag food for clients, you can designate volunteers as co-shoppers, not to serve as the food police, but to make conversation and interact with guests. If the volunteers have the same routine shift (say Tuesday afternoons), then they can get to know the same guests and learn about their situations and their families. In addition to providing food, food pantries can be opportune settings for people to feel seen and heard and to connect with others, particularly those outside their social circle, so they feel less alone.

These interactions between guests, volunteers, and staff can build social capital. Robert Putnam, a professor at Harvard, describes social capital in his book *Bowling Alone* and on his website as the benefits that flow from the trust, reciprocity, information, and cooperation associated with social networks. The cool thing about social capital is that it is a community asset—the guests will benefit but so too will the volunteers and staff who develop meaningful relationships with guests.

Connection creates a positive ripple effect. Just as a screwdriver (physical capital) or an education (human capital) makes us more productive, the connections we build through social capital can improve our health and well-being.

A Welcoming Culture with Customer Service

Dave Reed, the agency relations coordinator at the Worcester County Food Bank in Massachusetts, used to work at Starbucks. He describes how when someone is hired as a new barista, they are not just trained to use the register, they learn about customer service and hospitality, how to handle unhappy customers, and how to make customers feel welcome. He created a workshop to train food pantry staff and volunteers about these soft skills. Just as food bank staff provide trainings on food safety, it is also important to provide trainings on hospitality and customer service. He encourages food pantry directors to think of the "flow" of their pantry, from when people enter to how they shop. Consider what the experience is like when people come to get help.

Dave discusses ways to reduce barriers for people to receive help, from language barriers to organizational barriers such as cumbersome paperwork and eligibility requirements. Following are some additional things to consider to reduce stigma and improve the culture of a food pantry setting.

Reduction in Wait Times

Think about the experience of the guests who come to receive food at a food pantry. Are the lines and distribution systems set up to ease stress or do they add to the stress? If someone has experienced trauma, invading their personal space can feel threatening. Having to stand close to others while waiting in line can trigger anxiety. Is the pantry only open for a two-hour window, which can be stressful if the bus runs late? Does the food sometimes run out, so people are encouraged to line up early to make sure they get food?

These long lines create tension and stigma, hurting clients' self-esteem. Try to make the wait time for food as short and as comfortable as possible. Provide seats for people who are waiting and water and coffee if possible. I know what you may be thinking—we don't have enough space or time or volunteers or supplies to avoid long lines. This is the scarcity mentality at work. Even on a tight budget, small changes or reallocation of resources can create dramatic improvements.

In my experience, the food pantries that have the longest wait times are the ones that are open the shortest amount of time on the fewest days of the week.

In my experience, the food pantries that have the longest wait times are the ones that are open the shortest amount of time on the fewest days of the week. If your pantry is open on Tuesday mornings from 10 a.m. to 12 p.m., people probably start lining up around 7 a.m. Your volunteers will be hustling, and the whole operation will feel like a fire drill.

Is it possible for you to stay open for more hours or days of the week to reduce the frenzy and serve people without long wait times, giving them more time to shop in the pantry? Is it possible for you to redesign your space to allow for a waiting area with seats? Discuss strategies you can take to ensure that there will always be enough food and a good variety of food for those you serve. Food banks may provide capacity building grants to help food pantries open additional days of the week or evening and weekend hours or to help pay for chairs in a waiting area.

Spoiler alert: At the end of the book I advocate for consolidating smaller pantries to pool resources of volunteers, space, equipment, and funding. You may not have enough resources as a separate food pantry to reduce wait times, but if you work with other pantries you probably do. This will help create more holistic food pantries that can serve guests multiple days of the week while avoiding long lines and providing more dignity and wraparound services.

Sometimes a solution doesn't require additional funding but just some creativity. At Grace Episcopal Church in Hartford, Connecticut, food pantry clients used to wait in a long line outside the church and down the sidewalk before every pantry distribution on Thursday mornings. Recognizing that this was not the most dignified way to serve their guests, the pantry director opened the church and invited people to come sit inside in the pews. Guests receive a number and then can sit wherever they want in the church while they wait to shop. The pantry is still open only one day a week, but the directors found that the mood and atmosphere improved dramatically.

Lottery System

Another option to reduce wait times and to discourage guests from arriving hours before the distribution starts is to use a lottery system when handing out numbers. It is not a first-come-first-served system but rather a way to create equity and fairness. The Oregon Food Bank describes how their lottery system "helps make sure that everyone has an equal chance to shop, even if they can't always get to the pantry first because of their transportation, work schedule, or other circumstances."

Here is how it works. When the distribution is about to start, staff or volunteers determine how many people are in line and they shuffle that amount of numbers in a container. They hand out numbers that are randomly drawn from the container and then start with one. In this way, everyone has a chance to shop but the order changes with each distribution. You will want to communicate this change to guests in advance, and even with preparation, you may encounter frustration. Yet several programs have found success with this approach.

Ellie Nedry, senior community programs manager at the Second Harvest Food Bank of Orange County, has found a lottery works well for her Senior Grocery program. Before using the lottery system, one pantry had seniors arriving earlier and earlier, waiting out in the sun. The heat became a safety issue during the summer months, and it was impossible for some of the seniors to stand in line so long. The seniors were very resistant to the lottery system at first but have since adjusted, and now no line forms hours in advance.

Zane Hatfield at the Yolo Food Bank described how at their larger distributions they "encountered people sleeping in their cars overnight to ensure first place in line." They implemented a lottery system whereby about thirty minutes before the distribution starts, numbers are handed out in random order. It has prevented people from showing up extra early.

Physical Space

Think about the entrance to the pantry where guests arrive. Make sure there are clear, visible signs that display the name of your pantry and your days and hours of operation. Avoid confusion and misunderstandings by providing clear and accurate information. The signs and materials should include translations in the languages spoken by your guests. Make sure the physical space, including bathrooms and hallways, are well lit. Standing in a dark hallway does not feel safe. Think about the last time you painted the walls. Are the walls a drab grey? A fresh coat of paint doesn't cost a lot and can do wonders for how your space feels. Posting artwork or inspirational quotes on the walls can create a welcoming atmosphere. Have chairs available for people to sit and interact with one another. If possible, create a space for children to play.

In traditional food pantries, a wall may separate clients waiting for food from volunteers bagging the food. It is hard to make connections and build relationships when volunteers and clients do not share space or interact. Breaking down physical barriers leads to breaking down emotional ones as well. Providing a comfortable place for guests to interact while they wait to shop can reinforce a sense of community, helping guests feel connected, less alone, and more able to support one another.

Barrier Reduction

Think about the information you collect from guests as part of your intake process and why you need it. This is important and sets the tone for your program. Gathering information to determine if someone is poor, such as pay stubs, or to verify how many people live in a household, such as birth certificates, is intrusive and will discourage people from seeking help. As much as possible, we want to reduce these barriers. Can you simplify your process to make it easier and less stigmatizing for people to access your services?

Think about how much time your staff and volunteers spend on the intake process to check people in. Could this time be better spent on other activities? Think about how much sensitive or confidential information you collect and if it is necessary. What is the minimum amount of information needed to identify your clients? Is the rationale for collecting the information to make sure people don't take more food than others or visit your pantry too frequently? Creating an environment that is welcoming and dignified starts with trusting that if people are coming for help, they need the food. Focusing less on fraud and more on building trust will create a better experience not just for your guests but for your staff and volunteers too.

Most food pantries limit how frequently guests can shop for food and limit their services to a certain geographic area because they don't have unlimited resources. This is reasonable and makes sense. But besides name and address, what other information do you really need to know? If you want to help enroll guests in additional social service programs such as SNAP or utility assistance, they will need to provide much more detailed information, but you can do that in a private setting once they've expressed an interest in applying for the program.

Stressful Situations

Tensions can run high at food pantries. People are more likely to act out when they feel they are losing power, losing respect, or being shamed. But even when we try our best to create a calm and welcoming space, people can become upset. We want to be prepared with tools for dealing with stressful situations. Social service providers or public health agencies can provide trauma-informed care trainings for food pantry staff. At Foodshare, we invited a community partner to provide a de-escalation training for our staff, and we plan to offer the training for our partner programs. We recognized strains at our mobile food pantry program and realized that our staff could use some strategies for reducing the stress level.

The trainer gave practical tips for reflective listening, such as reflecting back what a guest says and identifying the feeling being expressed. He also offered suggestions for remaining calm and validating the guest's concerns. Rather than simply saying "these are our rules," we can acknowledge that the person feels frustrated and then explain that we want to make sure we can serve everyone. If someone is getting angry, listen carefully to what she or he is saying. Show empathy and validate their concerns. You can let guests know that you hear them (even if you don't agree with them) and that you care. For example: "I hear that you wanted to get meat today. I get how frustrating it is not to get it, and I wish I had it to give to you." "I hear that you'd like to get more corn. I wish we could give you more, but we need to make sure we have enough for everyone today." Just knowing that someone is listening can de-escalate someone's anger.

*Envision a food pantry
that is designed to be less
of a transaction and more
of a transformation of
lives and attitudes.*

The importance of creating a dignified culture at a food pantry and building relationships between staff, volunteers, and guests cannot be overstated. The food may be the reason why people come to a food pantry, but social interactions and the resulting connections can be a factor that helps them get back on their feet and not need to go to the food pantry long-term. Envision a food pantry that is designed to be less of a transaction and more of a transformation of lives and attitudes. This can be a simple interaction to help put a smile on someone's face and brighten someone's day or a deeper and longer-lasting transformation that comes through relationships and helping someone set and achieve goals in their life.

The Example of House of Hope

I have had the privilege of visiting a model food pantry in Stuart, Florida, called House of Hope. As the pantry has expanded over the years, the staff has redesigned its layout and processes. When you walk in the door, there is an inviting waiting area and front desk. Comfortable chairs are available, the space is painted in bright colors, and inspiring quotes appear on the walls. Staff at the front desk are friendly and either register new guests or check in existing guests.

House of Hope is open Monday through Friday and because people usually have appointment times, there is little wait time. Volunteers are available to assist, but guests pick out their own food. Glass-front refrigerators make it easy to see available fresh produce and dairy items. I discuss food choice in more detail in the next chapter, but this pantry has taken an extra step that is worth noting here. When guests finish shopping, they go to a counter that looks very much like a grocery store checkout except there obviously isn't a cash register. When I spoke with the director about this, he said that the staff intentionally designed the pantry to look and feel like a grocery store so that guests would not feel embarrassed. Children shopping with parents may not even notice a difference. The pantry is designed to reduce stigma. This speaks to the culture of the organization.

Thinking of the little details can make a huge difference in the guest experience. Yes, it helps that House of Hope has several paid staff, they are open multiple days a week, and the director is a savvy fundraiser. They are an example of a community food hub. But regardless of your budget or size, I hope this chapter offers ideas for how you can create a welcoming environment in your own food pantry. Creating a friendly, trauma-informed, and dignified culture requires staff and volunteers at all levels to understand these values and incorporate them into their day-to-day interactions with the people they serve.

Action Steps

- At the food bank, provide trainings on de-escalation and trauma-informed care for your staff and your partner programs, including food pantries.
- Provide workshops on customer service and hospitality; you can check out trainings by hotel chains such as Hilton.
- Create comfortable places to sit. Set up a waiting area with toys and books.
- Paint the walls a new cheerful color and hang artwork or inspirational quotes on the walls.
- Designate a "greeter" whose main job is to welcome people to the pantry.
- Provide fresh coffee and tea while people wait.
- If you have a large distribution and a wait time of over thirty minutes, consider using a lottery system to discourage people from showing up too early.

- Install a TV monitor displaying information about your programs or quotes from previous clients.

Are you starting to make changes? I thought so.

Resources

Brown, Brené. *Dare to Lead.* New York: Random House, 2018.

Corbett, Steve, and Brian Fikkert. *When Helping Hurts: How to Alleviate Poverty without Hurting the Poor . . . and Yourself.* Chicago: Moody Publishers, 2012.

de Souza, Rebecca. *Feeding the Other: Whiteness, Privilege and Neoliberal Stigma in Food Pantries.* Cambridge, MA: MIT Press, 2019.

Guarino, Kathleen, Phoebe Soares, Kristina Konnath, Rose Clervil, and Ellen Bassuk. *Trauma-Informed Organizational Toolkit.* Rockville, MD: Center for Mental Health Services, Substance Abuse and Mental Health Services Administration, and the Daniels Fund, the National Child Traumatic Stress Network, and the W. K. Kellogg Foundation, 2009. https://www.air.org/sites/default/files/downloads/report/Trauma-Informed_Organizational_Toolkit_0.pdf.

Gunderson, Craig, Emily Engelhard, and Monica Hake. "The Determinants of Food Insecurity among Food Bank Clients in the United States." *Journal of Consumer Affairs* 51, no. 3 (2017): 501–518. https://doi.org/10.1111/joca.12157.

Lupton, Robert. *Toxic Charity: How Churches and Charities Hurt Those They Help (And How to Reverse It).* New York: HarperOne, 2011.

Martin, Katie, Beatrice Rogers, John Cook, and Hugh Joseph. "Social Capital Is Associated with Decreased Risk of Hunger." *Social Science & Medicine* 58, no. 12 (2004): 2645–2654. https://doi.org/10.1016/j.socscimed.2003.09.026.

Putnam, Robert. Social Capital Primer. http://robertdputnam.com/bowling-alone/social-capital-primer/.

Seligman, Hilary K., and Dean Schillinger. "Hunger and Socioeconomic Disparities in Chronic Disease." *New England Journal of Medicine* 363, no. 1 (July 2010): 6–9. https://doi.org/10.1056/NEJMp1000072.

CHAPTER 5
The Dignity of Choice

Imagine going to a restaurant and rather than giving you a menu, the waiter simply brings you a meal. Or going to the grocery store and instead of shopping for your family, being handed two bags of food. Unfortunately, this is how traditional food pantries operate. Now there is a chance that you might be pleasantly surprised by the food in the bags or enjoy the convenience. But you might also be disappointed because your family doesn't eat those particular foods or they're not what you need at the moment. Maybe you already have two jars of peanut butter at home and what you really need is rice and beans.

Providing people with the dignity to select their own food at a food pantry is an important first step in creating an environment that helps people help themselves. Allowing people to choose their food, what is called "client choice" or "customer choice," helps create an empowering setting. Whether you take this step says a lot about the mission and values of a food pantry.

In the last chapter, I discussed the importance of creating an environment that is trauma informed. For someone who has experienced trauma, a sense of control is vital, even when that control is over something as simple as a food selection. In short, choice builds confidence and self-esteem.

Traditional Food Distribution

For years, most food pantries have been designed and operated so that food is collected and stored in one area of the pantry and volunteers come to sort, organize, and prepare bags of food for clients in advance. Clients are told to wait their turn in line, and when they reach the front of the line, they are handed the prepacked bags of food. This system tends to work very well for volunteers, and the roles are clearly defined. Volunteers handle and organize the food, perhaps give people numbers indicating their place in the queue, and hand out food. It seems efficient because during distribution you can serve a large number of people quickly and you know everyone is getting the same type and amount of food.

But here's the problem. This system is not best for the people we are serving, the customers. I'll give a few examples to show the downsides of this approach. Then I'll provide compelling reasons to allow more choice and practical steps for converting pantries to a choice model.

Unintended Consequences

At Foodshare, we recently received complaints from a few clients who attended one of our member food pantries, saying they were treated unfairly. Our agency relations staff member went to observe for herself how the program was operated. Sure enough, as people waited in line, one of the volunteers was rather rude to clients, telling them to stay in line, and if they made a comment about the wait or the food they received, the volunteer quipped, "Hey, this isn't Stop & Shop" (a local grocery store chain in New England, and for those of you in other parts of the country, you can insert Kroger, Wegmans, Giant, Piggly Wiggly, or your local chain). In this situation, clients do not have choice; instead, the message is that they should be grateful to receive whatever is handed to them. In other words, beggars can't be choosers. My friends, we can do better.

The Ohio Association of Second Harvest Food Banks created a great manual that describes how and why to make the switch to client choice, and I've included a link in the resource list at the end of the chapter. The manual explains, "While traditional pantry clients may present a demeanor of gratitude for the service, you can rest assured that they are not proud of having a box of pre-selected food handed to them. Add to this the public stigma of relying on food pantries in the first place, and it becomes apparent that providing a single point of flexibility (in this case, personal food choice) will have a significantly positive impact on the client's confidence level." Offering customer choice can go a long way toward decreasing the stigma and sometimes humiliation of going to a food pantry.

Food Waste

Food banks were created to help provide food for those in need and to reduce food waste. It seems like a great dual mission. Traditional food pantries may seem efficient in terms of moving food quickly, but they are often not efficient from the standpoint of food waste. When volunteers put food into everyone's bags, then everyone receives the same food whether they want it

At food pantries where there is no choice, you may see clients trading food with other clients, leaving food items in the parking lot, or throwing food away once they get home.

or not. At food pantries where there is no choice, you may see clients trading food with other clients, leaving food items in the parking lot, or throwing food away once they get home. This is wasteful and certainly not what the program intended.

A food pantry director once told me a humorous yet sad story to explain why she decided to switch to client choice. She routinely ordered some specific items from the food bank that cannot be found at a grocery store. Their labels have a distinct brand name and look that makes them easy to identify. The pantry held a local food drive, and someone donated one of these food bank items. The only way this could happen was for a client to receive it from the pantry, then donate it back to the pantry. Talk about defeating the purpose of providing charitable food! This was a stark wake-up call that if the client had the option to choose their food, they would never have selected this item.

Recently I talked with a food pantry staff member in Massachusetts who admitted he had been skeptical about allowing people to choose their food. But once his pantry made the switch, he saw how choice increased efficiency. Beforehand, clients used to discard food that they didn't want at the end of the distribution line, and volunteers had to re-shelve it. Afterwards, the flow of the pantry line ran more smoothly.

Examples from No Choice, Limited Choice, to Full Choice

When I ask food pantry directors if they allow clients to choose their food, the vast majority will say yes. I have heard some food bank staff members say that all of the food pantries in their network are choice pantries. But just like most practices within food pantry settings, there are varying degrees of client choice, and they matter. Remember, it's important not to think about these strategies as one-size-fits-all, or as "all or nothing." For example, either you offer client choice or you don't.

Rather, it is helpful to understand the different ways and levels of providing choice so staff can see how they might design their pantry differently and make small changes to improve services.

I've already described a traditional pantry that has no choice, where each client is given a prepacked bag or box to take home. A next step is providing prepacked bags of food and then having a "choice" table with a few items that people can select, often at the end of the line. This is a very limited way of offering choice, and the selection on the choice table is often of mediocre quality. Next along the continuum would be providing a list of food items, like a menu, for clients to choose. Then volunteers take the selected list and go to another room to pack the food. For example, a client might select soup, tuna, and pasta. Clients may not be able to select the different types of soup or pasta, but they have some choice of food items. Similarly, other food pantries ask clients to stand behind a counter so they can see the food and tell volunteers which items they want, but volunteers do the bagging.

My simple definition of customer choice is that guests get to touch and select their own food. Period. To me, if someone else is physically selecting and handing the food to clients, then there isn't full choice.

My simple definition of customer choice is that guests get to touch and select their own food. Period. To me, if someone else is physically selecting and handing the food to clients, then there isn't full choice. If guests do not actually touch their food, this is still a limited or modified version of choice.

Feeding America describes the various points on the spectrum of choice, starting with a "choice food pantry" that offers fully open shopping with no limits; a pantry that allows beneficiaries to select the foods they want off the shelf, with limits on the amounts of different items; or a pantry where beneficiaries point and tell the individual who is packing the box what they want, within the limits of each item. The common denominator is that food is not distributed as prepacked items selected by someone besides the beneficiary. The variables depend on how the choice is made and with what limitations.

Full Customer Choice

The best scenario is when guests can walk through the pantry, touch the food, and select their own items off the shelves. Volunteers may play an assistant role, simply describing how many items a family can take. The volunteers can then spend more time talking with guests, asking about their family, maybe sharing recipes and helping guests to select healthy options. If space allows, it is best to set up the pantry like a small grocery store with grocery carts for guests to load their food. But even with limited space, you can allow guests to pick their food from shelves or tables. Any type of food pantry can offer choice.

Giving people choice does not mean allowing them to take as much as they want. Almost all food pantries, regardless of choice, set limits on how much food guests can select. Food pantries usually display signs that explain how many items can be selected for each food group, sometimes with a sliding scale by family size, and this is often determined by how much food is available at the pantry. For example, you can take two cans of vegetables, one box of pasta, one jar of peanut butter, and so on. But with choice, the guests can select the items they want (choosing canned peas instead of carrots) or choose not to take an item that they don't want or need. If a guest already has enough tuna at home, they often feel better leaving the tuna for others to take. If a guest is disabled, elderly, or otherwise impaired, volunteers can certainly help select food and carry bags. But the default should be to allow people to choose their food.

Even though client choice is nationally recognized as a best practice, surprisingly it is not standardized or even routinely practiced in food pantry settings. We can do better.

When we think about client choice pantries, we tend to include limited and modified versions of choice in our definition and therefore may not recognize the opportunity to expand to full choice. A recent study by Christopher Long from the University of Arkansas and his colleagues evaluated over 350 food pantries in Arkansas within five food bank networks. They found that only 19 percent of pantries offered client choice. From my experience, many food pantry directors, and some food bank staff, have not seen many other food pantries and may not appreciate the benefits of offering client choice. Raising awareness of the different levels of choice is an important first step.

Even though client choice is nationally recognized as a best practice, surprisingly it is not standardized or even routinely practiced in food pantry settings. We can do better.

The Breaking Down of Barriers

These changes may seem trivial. Why does this matter? Why am I making such a big deal about how food is distributed when the end goal is making sure people have food? When there are so many people in need, shouldn't we just focus on getting food to them, any food, as quickly as possible? And if people really don't have enough food to eat, shouldn't they simply be grateful for the food they are given? Trust me, I've heard these questions before.

Not giving guests the ability to choose their food sends an understated message of distrust. This messaging is clearly out of sync with our goal of helping people help themselves. We can't expect people to enroll in a job training program, or change their eating habits, or enroll in SNAP if we don't trust them to choose their own food. When we set up barriers, such as a counter or wall, between guests and the food they will take home, with volunteers as the gatekeepers, we reinforce the power dynamic of giver and receiver. By preparing bags of food in advance, we are putting the convenience of volunteers ahead of the needs of our guests. When volunteers select the food, it also creates an emotional barrier between the volunteers and clients. The volunteers are in charge and the clients are at their mercy.

This is important. Even if well intentioned, these barriers create divisions and limit our ability to build relationships. Think about how you like to shop for your food and the choices you are able to make. It's easy to take these things for granted. Hopefully you can appreciate the subtle yet important differences between the various models of choice. Understanding these distinctions provides opportunities for growth. Are the pantries in your food bank network operating at the full level of choice or using only a modified version? Can you describe these differences and help your programs make additional changes? You can use this information to help nudge your pantries toward full choice.

> *When we set up barriers, such as a counter or wall, between guests and the food they will take home, with volunteers as the gatekeepers, we reinforce the power dynamic of giver and receiver.*

Benefits of Offering Customer Choice

A few examples of the benefits of giving people the opportunity to choose their own food include the following:

- Reduces waste because guests will not receive items that they do not want, need, or have the ability to use

- Encourages a dignified experience in which guests feel respected by the staff and volunteers
- Makes it easier to order food that is desired by guests and culturally sensitive to guests' needs
- Provides an opportunity for pantries to tailor food items and sections of the pantry to address guests' health needs, for example, designing a diabetes-friendly section
- Reduces stigma because the shopping experience feels more like going to a grocery store than receiving charity
- Allows more interactions between guests, volunteers, and staff so they can get to know one another better

The recent study by Long and colleagues of over 350 food pantries in Arkansas found that pantries offering choice served more healthy food items than nonchoice pantries. The Akron–Canton Regional Foodbank in Ohio found that the client choice system can require fewer staff and volunteer hours since the bags are packed as clients come in and choose their food. And as the staff become familiar with popular food items, they can spend less money ordering unpopular ones. Compared with standard prepacked bags, they found that client choice can cost less to operate.

Most of the evidence about the benefits of client choice is anecdotal—stories we hear from food pantry directors and guests. More research is needed to evaluate the impact on client outcomes when a pantry converts from handing out prepacked bags to allowing guests to choose their food. Research should focus on outcomes such as increased food security and diet quality, but also on emotional health and well-being. Some research questions worth exploring include

- Do guests feel less stigma and feel more comfortable shopping at a choice pantry compared with nonchoice pantries?

- Do customers waste less food and make fewer trade-off decisions (between food, rent, and medicine) when shopping at a choice pantry compared with nonchoice pantries?

If we find significant differences, which I hypothesize we will, we can use the results to encourage additional pantries to offer full choice. While hard data is important, so too is the experience of individual pantries and their guests. One encouraging example comes from a food pantry in Westerly, Rhode Island, called the Jonnycake Center. It's a wonderful pantry with a social service office, a thrift store, and other wraparound services for guests. I visited the pantry a few years ago. The pantry enjoys a very large space with organized rows of shelving to store food. However, it offered very little choice. Clients would sit in a waiting area and fill out a form to select food, and the volunteers would go to the other side of a wall to put the food into bags for the clients. I described the importance of choice and suggested that they allow clients to come "behind the wall" to select their own food. Space was not an issue; they just hadn't thought about client choice in this way before.

"My parents struggled with pride because they worked. Pride can stop people from getting help. When you're handed a bag of food it is belittling."

I'm happy to say that they renovated their space to allow for full client choice. One of their customers told me, "I choose things I would actually eat. They are giving people power back." She continued, "My parents struggled with pride because they worked. Pride can stop people from getting help. When you're handed a bag of food it is belittling."

Concerns about Offering Choice

You may think you cannot provide client choice in your pantry. Trust me, you can and you should. I recognize that there may be challenges.

I've heard many reasons why converting to client choice would be hard. There are subtle fears and worries at the heart of delivering food in traditional food pantry models. Human beings in general don't like change. These are common concerns with allowing clients to choose their food:

- There isn't enough space to allow for people to choose.
- It will take too much time.
- Clients will take too much food.
- This is how we've always operated our food pantry, and the volunteers won't like change.

But here is the thing, from my experience talking to many food bank staff and food pantry directors over the years, when food pantries shift to client choice, 100 percent of the time people say it has worked well. One hundred percent of the time. I'm not kidding—it's an amazing track record. They say it is a better experience for their guests and for their volunteers, and they wish they had done it sooner. It is simply a better way to design and operate a food pantry.

Table Distributions

If pantries do not have permanent space or equipment to design the pantry like a grocery store, they may set up tables during the food distributions. Volunteers bring the food from storage and place it onto tables, and then customers walk by the tables to select their food. Even in pantries that have quick distributions serving many people, even when there isn't a lot of variety in the selection of food, and there are just a few items that everyone will receive, I say to you: let people touch and choose their own food.

I witnessed this in a small church pantry that for years had volunteers prebag all of their food. Then they switched to "choice," but all this meant was that food was set out on tables and when clients walked through the line, they received a different food item from each volunteer at each table. There really wasn't any choice involved. Everyone still got the same food, but now they walked through a line to have food placed in their bags by the same volunteers who used to bag the food in advance.

The unwritten, subtle instructions for clients were to walk through the line with their hand out. Not very empowering. We often talk symbolically about wanting to provide not just a handout but a hand up. But if we are selecting food for clients, and asking them to put their hand out to receive it, we are not fulfilling our greater mission.

> *We often talk symbolically about wanting to provide not just a handout but a hand up. But if we are selecting food for clients, and asking them to put their hand out to receive it, we are not fulfilling our greater mission.*

I suggested that the volunteers simply stand behind the table and tell clients how many items they could choose. Guests were so accustomed to holding their bag out to get the food that it was a little awkward at first. Yet some people smiled and seemed to appreciate being able to select their own food. Volunteers were so accustomed to quickly placing a food item in each person's bag that it was awkward for them too. Several people chose not to take a food item, either because they didn't care for it or they already had enough of it at home. This seemed liberating for guests to be able to say no or make a choice between items.

I also suggested that the food pantry director set out a couple of different options for each category when possible. Because the pantry allowed people to shop once a week, the director tried to mix up the options and provide canned corn one week, then green beans the next week, then carrots. I suggested she try to offer a few different options each week and let people make their own selections. This was more work for the volunteers because they had to track more items each week, but it provided more variety and choice for guests. The pantry director noticed people liked this change, and then she could find out which items people preferred and order more of those.

I have witnessed the effects of no choice, limited choice, and full client choice. Trust me, it makes a difference. If we are serious about helping people, not just with food for today, but to get back on their feet and become self-sufficient, then we need to allow them to choose their food. It builds the foundation for the other important changes we will discuss in the next few chapters. It starts with choice.

The Conversion to Client Choice

So how does a traditional food pantry make the switch to client choice? Think about the space you currently use to have volunteers sort and bag food. If you currently use large tables, consider replacing this space with shelves. You will save space because you will have more vertical room to store food. Many metal shelves have wheels so you can physically move them around if need be when the pantry is not open. If your pantry currently has a large space used for storage, you can add shelves and create aisles for shopping. Use the space to organize food onto shelves where people can select their food directly from the shelf, rather than to simply store your food. It's great if there is room for extra storage, and then shelves for shopping, but even small closets can be designed to allow people to choose their food. Remember, any space can be used to offer choice.

When a pantry converts to choice, how and when volunteers spend their time will change. If the pantry is open only a limited number of days each month and you are serving many people at each distribution, it may seem impossible to allow people to choose their own food because it will take too much time. You may need to consider opening your pantry on additional days or times to spread out the times when people shop. You can start by utilizing the time that volunteers would have spent simply preparing bags. This will require different roles for volunteers or a different schedule for when you are open. If volunteers spend two hours preparing bags and then two hours distributing bags, that is four hours total that could be used for guests to shop. Those four hours might be used for one longer day of shopping or perhaps might be spread over a couple of different days.

The volunteer experience will change too. While you will still need volunteers to help load food onto shelves and organize the pantry, more time can be spent interacting with customers rather than the mundane task of loading food items into dozens of bags. The underlying goal of our charitable food programs is not simply to provide food but to provide a dignified experience in which people can select the food they want and need. Another goal is to provide a meaningful experience for volunteers as well. To make these types of transitions, volunteer training is often required to explain why this type of change will improve the pantry and how the changes will be made.

> *While you will still need volunteers to help load food onto shelves and organize the pantry, more time can be spent interacting with customers rather than the mundane task of loading food items into dozens of bags.*

Think about the layout of your current space and consider how shoppers come through your pantry. Can you reconfigure the space or move some furniture into different positions to create a better flow? Get creative. Ideally, you can set up the pantry like a small grocery store with shopping carts. Ask your food bank for referrals to other food pantries in your area that are full choice and go see how they are designed. A manual from Ohio food banks that provides tangible descriptions for converting to choice is included in the resource list at the end of the chapter.

Because every food pantry operates a little differently, it is important to be clear about the different ways that pantries offer choice. Understanding the different types of choice models can provide steps and goals for increasing choice over time. If a pantry currently offers prepacked bags, it may be intimidating to convert to full choice. Starting with modified or limited choice can be a transitional step.

Suggested Equipment

These are suggestions for the types of equipment needed when providing client choice:

- Shelves to organize and display food
- Display signs with clear information and pretty pictures
- Shopping carts
- Reusable bags—encourage guests to bring their own
- Refrigerators

We recommend glass-front refrigerators so guests can see the food inside. If you need help purchasing a fridge, talk with your food bank or local donors for support. A staff member at Foodshare has a friend who works for Coca-Cola, and that company replaces their refrigerators frequently in retail stores. Several refrigerators have been donated to our local partner programs simply because she asked.

The Vermont Foodbank created an awesome Pinterest page and Instagram page with links to various bins and storage items to help display fresh fruits and vegetables as part of their VT Fresh program. They provide a lot of inspiration for designing choice pantries that look more like Whole Foods groceries than nonperishable food closets.

If you receive food from local food drives, you can encourage people to donate specific food items that you have a hard time sourcing from the food bank and which are popular with your guests. For example, you can ask for a cereal drive (preferably low-sugar options) or a peanut butter drive. Not only will you stock more food that your guests like, but it will be easier to organize on your shelves for when guests come to shop.

One last pitch about customer choice. One of the best examples of providing people who are food insecure with the dignity to choose their own food is through SNAP. The first line of defense against hunger, SNAP is the best way to ensure that people can select their own food. In addition to providing choice in the food pantry, it is also important to provide information about SNAP and help people enroll in the program so they can shop for food at the grocery store.

Action Steps

- If you work at a food bank, gather information from your pantries to determine their level of choice. I provide a measurement tool for this in chapter 9. Then provide trainings and resources to build the capacity of your pantries to offer additional levels of choice.
- Encourage traditional food pantries to visit client choice pantries to see how they operate. Celebrate food pantries that offer full choice as role models in your community.
- If you work at or volunteer at a pantry, talk with the director about client choice. Rearrange the shelves to allow for choice. Discuss and reassign the roles of volunteers. Talk with your guests about this switch in operations. Set a time frame and let volunteers and guests know when you will be changing your operations.
- Reassign roles for your food pantry volunteers and modify days and times when guests can shop to allow for more choice.
- Think about the amount of time and energy the volunteers spend preparing bags of food. Reallocate this volunteer time to time when guests can shop at the pantry. Volunteers can spend some of their time to organize the shelves, but the majority of their time should be with the guests to greet them, get to know them, share stories about favorite recipes, and build relationships.
- Make one change to offer more choice for your customers. We all like to have choices in life.

Resources

Long, Christopher, Marie-Rachelle Narcisse, Brett Rowland, Bonnie Faitak, Caitlin Caspi, Joel Gittelsohn, and Pearl McElfish. "Written Nutrition Guidelines, Client Choice Distribution, and Adequate Refrigerator Storage Are Positively Associated with Increased Offerings of Feeding America's Detailed Foods to Encourage (F2E) in a Large Sample of Arkansas Food Pantries." *Journal of the Academy of Nutrition and Dietetics* 120, no. 5 (2019): 792–803. https://doi.org/10.1016/j.jand.2019.08.017.

Ohio Association of Second Harvest Food Banks. *Making the Switch: A Guide for Converting to a Client Choice Food Pantry.* http://site.foodshare.org/site/DocServer/Making_the_Switch_to_Client_Choice.pdf?docID=6081.

Stluka, Suzanne, Lindsay Moore, Heather Eicher-Miller, Lisa Franzen-Castle, Becky Henne, Donna Mehrle, Daniel Remley, and Lacey McCormack. "Voices for Food: Methodologies for Implementing a Multi-state Community-based Intervention in Rural, High Poverty Communities." *BMC Public Health* 18, no. 1 (2018): 1055. https://doi.org/10.1186/s12889-018-5957-9.

University of Minnesota Extension. "Building Better Food Shelves." https://extension.umn.edu/nutrition-and-healthy-eating/building-better-food-shelves.

Vermont Foodbank. "VT Fresh." https://www.instagram.com/vtfreshprogram/.

CHAPTER 6

Promotion of Healthy Food

In the early 1980s when most food banks were started, we didn't have a national obesity epidemic, and we didn't see the connection between hunger and health. Food banks and food pantries were focused on people not having enough food, and the logical response was to provide food, regardless of its nutritional quality. In terms of food donations, the goal was, and often continues to be, to provide calorie-dense, shelf-stable, and nonperishable food to fill hungry bellies. When I started doing antihunger work in the early 1990s, I would say, "I'm worried about whether people have *enough* food, I'm not worried about the quality of the food." Wow, how things have changed. Hopefully this chapter shows how "calories are not just calories," because there is a preponderance of evidence showing the link between food insecurity and food-related chronic diseases.

In this chapter, I provide data about the strong connection between hunger and health, discuss ways to promote healthy food in food pantries, describe the value of nutrition policies and nutrition ranking systems, and provide suggestions for moving beyond canned food drives.

But first, let's be clear about the relationship between food insecurity and chronic diseases.

Obesity Epidemic

In the United States, rising obesity rates became a concern during the 1980s and have been attributed to a host of economic, social, and political factors. For example, beginning in the mid-1970s, the federal government changed decades of agricultural policy and began providing direct subsidies to farmers to grow a few specific crops, including corn and soybeans, which were then made into very inexpensive ingredients such as high fructose corn syrup and vegetable oil. These cheap raw ingredients are used to create many highly processed, inexpensive, yet highly caloric products such as soda, snacks, and desserts. For a great historical description of these trends, I highly recommend Michael Pollan's book *The Omnivore's Dilemma*. Other trends that contribute to obesity include increases in fast food and convenient meals, increased use of technology, and more sedentary lifestyles, among others.

When data started to emerge in the 1990s that people who were food insecure were actually more likely to experience obesity, it was quite confusing. We used to call this the paradox of hunger with obesity.

When data started to emerge in the 1990s that people who were food insecure were actually more likely to experience obesity, it was quite confusing. We used to call this the *paradox* of hunger with obesity. It seemed illogical that you could not have enough money for food but at the same time become obese.

The food insecurity–obesity relationship is not surprising if you think about the relative cost of different grocery items. It is much easier to stretch your food dollar if you buy cheap, highly processed, calorie-dense foods. The types of foods that are recommended to prevent chronic diseases, such as fresh fruits and vegetables, low-fat dairy, lean meats, and whole grains tend to cost more than their less-healthy counterparts or require more time to prepare from scratch. They are also less likely to be available in low-income neighborhoods and communities of color. These factors make it difficult to access healthy food for your family if you are on a limited budget.

Like many topics discussed in this book, we still have work to do to shed light on this paradoxical relationship. Stereotypes and weight bias can limit our ability to help those in need. We typically think about hunger as undernutrition and lack of calories. But it is more appropriate to label hunger as malnutrition that can come from not enough calories or an overconsumption of cheap calories. It is important to dispel the myth that hunger and obesity cannot coexist. This is an example of why it is so important to keep up to date on the latest research and evidence, to evaluate the work we're doing, and to evolve our programming based on new information.

The Link between Hunger and Health

There is an incredible amount of research showing the strong connection between hunger and health and why we should focus not just on pounds of food but on the nutritional quality of charitable food. People who visit food pantries often have a double burden of food insecurity and chronic diseases, including both physical and mental health challenges. They are more likely to suffer from high blood pressure, high cholesterol, obesity, and heart disease. National data from the 2014 Hunger in America study found that among clients who visit food pantries, 58 percent of households had a member with high blood pressure and 33 percent had a member with diabetes. My colleagues and

I conducted a study of food pantry clients in Hartford, Connecticut, and we found similar results, showing that 65 percent had a household member with high blood pressure, and 26 percent had a household member with diabetes.

People struggling with food insecurity are also less likely to manage their disease well and more likely to have complications. Think about how many medications should be taken with food, which can be challenging when you do not have consistent access to it. Data from the 2014 Hunger in America study show that families struggling with food insecurity make difficult trade-off decisions, with 66 percent having to decide between paying for food and paying for medicine. One coping strategy used by the majority of households (79 percent) in the same study was to purchase inexpensive, unhealthy food to feed their family.

A food pantry client in Greater Hartford, Connecticut, sums up the dilemma well: "Food is expensive, and I've been buying basic things, because meat is expensive. I've been buying ramen noodle soup because it's cheap, but it's not healthy. When you have no income you eat unhealthy."

My colleagues Drs. Hilary Seligman from the University of California–San Francisco and Marlene Schwartz from the University of Connecticut Rudd Center for Food Policy and Obesity describe the missed opportunity of health professionals and food bank staff to make stronger connections between hunger and health. In a recent article in the *Journal of Hunger and Environmental Nutrition*, they write that food pantries are often overlooked as part of the food system. They say, "One reason is that nutrition and health researchers have lacked awareness of the size and scope—and therefore the potential importance—of the charitable feeding system. Another is that the system itself was focused on other priorities. The mission of food banks and food pantries is generally to end hunger (i.e., provide calories), not to improve nutrition, transform the food environment, or prevent diet-related illness."

Zip Codes and Food Access

Beyond the ability to afford healthy food, this is about access, and research shows that predominantly Black and Hispanic communities have fewer grocery stores and poorer quality food than predominantly White neighborhoods.

If you are food insecure, it can be challenging to buy healthy food, especially fresh fruits and vegetables. Low-income neighborhoods are often devoid of affordable and nutritious food, where people live more than a mile from a full-size supermarket in urban or suburban areas and over ten miles from a supermarket in rural areas. In urban areas, you may have a lot of highly processed, inexpensive, unhealthy food but limited supplies of healthy alternatives. Beyond the ability to afford healthy food, this is about access, and research shows that predominantly Black and Hispanic communities have fewer grocery stores and poorer quality food than predominantly White neighborhoods.

One of the most compelling statements that has recently emerged from the field of public health is that "your zip code is more important than your genetic code." Rather than our health being largely based on genes passed down from our ancestors, we know that much of our health rests in our socioeconomic status (our income, education, and employment status), the neighborhood in which we live, and what we have access to (including decent schools, jobs, and grocery stores). These are systemic inequalities. Research shows that people living in low-income zip codes can have significantly lower life expectancies than people living just a few miles away in a high-income zip code.

We live in an obesogenic environment—one that promotes overeating cheap calories and living sedentary lifestyles. An easy example is going to pay for your paint at the hardware store and encountering a full array of king-size candy bars that are two for $1. You came to buy paint but you leave with an extra 400 calories. It wasn't always this way. The food industry has made it very convenient and cheap to consume extra calories. And this toxic food environment is even more prevalent if you live in a low-income neighborhood that has few large supermarkets but many corner stores. We will likely need new regulations, modeled after restrictions on cigarettes, in order to reverse this trend and remove unhealthy food from checkouts. Just as advertisements for cigarettes are more common in low-income communities, so too are advertisements for fast food and junk food.

These issues may seem like a tangent from our discussion of charitable food, so let me connect the dots. When we understand that many families struggling with poverty and food insecurity also struggle with chronic diseases, and that low-income communities have very limited amounts of healthy, affordable food, then the need to provide healthy food in food banks and food pantries becomes obvious and more important. It is a matter of food justice. We must dispel the myth that people who are struggling with food insecurity prefer less nutritious food and are not interested in fruits and vegetables or other healthy items. Data don't support this notion.

Demand for Healthy Food

Often when I talk about promoting healthy food in food pantries, people will say how important it is to provide education. The subtle implication is that food pantry clients do not know what they should be eating or are making poor nutritional choices. It is true that nutrition education can be valuable, and I support partnering with nutrition educators to provide information and recipes in pantries. But quantitative and qualitative research has shown that food pantry clients already want to eat healthier food but often cannot afford it or find it in their local grocery stores or food pantries. Or the foods that are promoted are not familiar to them.

A few years ago when I was conducting surveys in a food pantry, I asked a client about the types of food he usually ate. He told me, "The doctor keeps telling me to eat more fruits and vegetables, and he doesn't know I can't afford them." The problem here is not just lack of knowledge or education but lack of access and affordability. In our early evaluation of the Freshplace food pantry in Hartford, Connecticut, we found significant improvements in fruit and vegetable consumption by the people who attended Freshplace compared with other traditional food pantries. As one Freshplace member said, "There are fresh vegetables that you don't normally get from the food pantry."

If you are on a limited budget in a low-income community, it is easy to find and afford highly processed food like chips, soda, and cookies, which contribute to chronic diseases. This is not what people are looking for when they go to a food pantry. My colleagues Drs. Marlene Schwartz and Kristen Cooksey-Stowers from the University of Connecticut and I conducted research to understand what food pantry guests in Connecticut *do* want to see at the pantry. The top five products were fruits and vegetables (70 percent), meats/fish (53 percent), 100 percent juice (41 percent), whole grain bread (41 percent), and dairy products (39 percent). The items at the bottom of the list were baby food (14 percent), regular soda (9 percent), and salty snacks (6 percent).

Cultural Food Availability

In addition to making healthy food available, it is key to pay attention to the cultural food preferences of the people we serve. I spoke with a registered dietitian who is working on a food is medicine program to provide medically tailored meals for people with chronic diseases. She said that she has been talking with her nutrition colleagues about the cultural appropriateness of the food they provide. For example, she said that most of her dietitian colleagues are White women, and they often promote items such as hummus, cottage cheese, and quinoa. Sure, these items are healthy, but they may not be familiar to people of color, let alone affordable or available. In fact, they may turn off the very people we are trying to serve. One strategy is to ask the people you serve what food items they are most interested in receiving or have them rank various

Ask your food pantry guests to provide their favorite recipes, and then ask a nutrition professional to tweak the recipe to be slightly healthier while maintaining the familiar cultural ingredients.

foods by preference. Ask your food pantry guests to provide their favorite recipes, and then ask a nutrition professional to tweak the recipe to be slightly healthier while maintaining the familiar cultural ingredients.

Susannah Morgan, the CEO of the Oregon Food Bank, describes how focusing on equity has changed their food bank in every way. It has changed the food that they buy. She explains that "when people think about equity they think about interpersonal relations. But it's about the way you see the world. Using an equity lens makes you slow down, see who is making decisions, what they might not know and who is not represented." Their food-purchasing staff used to buy a lot of tomato sauce. But this reflects cooking habits primarily of people from Northern Europe. By thinking about cultures with different dietary habits, they decided to use the same dollars to purchase diced tomatoes, which can be used for pasta sauce but also tacos, curry, and many other dishes.

Better Offerings than Beef Stew

I wonder how many people go to a food pantry looking specifically for beef stew. I admit this particular food is one of my pet peeves. It somehow became the poster child and seemingly requisite staple food

A typical food drive highlights the need for packaged, nonperishable food items and often the lists of requested food items are of questionable nutritional value, such as mac and cheese, stew, and pancake mix and syrup.

found in nearly every food pantry and food bank I've ever visited. The logic is that beef stew is a hearty, filling meal and therefore a necessary item for food insecure families. I'm curious, when was the last time you bought a can of beef stew to serve to your family? I'm guessing not very recently, yet somehow we think this is an important staple food item for our neighbors. While filling, one serving of beef stew typically contains enough sodium for a full day's recommended supply. It is like a heart attack in a can.

Recently, many food banks have received donations of beef stew from a government commodity program, and the beef stew is packaged in large aluminum pouches that look like something out of a sci-fi movie. These pouches are then provided for free to food pantries and offered to families. There is very little demand for the pouches because the stew is gelatinous and unappealing. This doesn't mean that we should only provide fruits and vegetables in food pantries, but there is much work to be done to increase access to healthy, appealing food within the charitable food system.

When we think about nutritional advice about maintaining good health, the basic tenets of a good diet include fruits, vegetables, whole grains, legumes, low-fat meat and dairy products, and food that is minimally processed. As Michael Pollan, who wrote *The Omnivore's Dilemma*, would say, "food that your grandmother would recognize." The less packaging, preservatives, and processing, the better for our health and that of our planet. Now think about solicitations from food pantries and food banks to help tackle hunger. A typical food drive highlights the need for packaged, nonperishable food items and often the lists of requested food items are of questionable nutritional value, such as mac and cheese, stew, and pancake mix and syrup. No wonder there is a disconnect between nutritional advice and health outcomes among food pantry clients. We can do better.

Nutrition Policies at Food Banks

As we think about the connection between hunger and health, it is important to understand the source of food donations. Food banks receive food from many sources, mainly from retail grocery stores and from food manufacturers, from the federal government through the Emergency Food Assistance Program and the Commodity Supplemental Food Program, and from local farmers. Much of this food is nonperishable, but food banks are also receiving more perishable items from retail stores and also co-op programs that provide bulk produce at discounts.

MAZON, a national advocacy organization working to end hunger, conducted a study in 2018 of food banks around the country and found that 25 percent of food distributed by food banks consisted of unhealthy beverages and snack foods. The authors argued that "meaningful progress to improve food quality in food banks is often stymied by food retailers, the largest donors to the charitable food system."

Even when staff at food banks are concerned about the nutritional quality of their food, they are often at the mercy of retail stores and manufacturers. I have heard many comments about not wanting to say no to a food donor, both from food bank and food pantry staff members. The argument is that we should be grateful for any food that is donated, and we run the risk of losing food or financial donations if we tell people what type of food we would like them to donate. This is scarcity mentality, and it seems quite defeatist. This is a missed opportunity.

One strategy for improving the nutritional quality of donated food (both at food banks and food pantries) is to enact a nutrition policy to highlight the strong connection between hunger and health, to describe the types of food that are most desirable, and to ban or request that donors not provide certain items, such as soda and candy. A nutrition policy can be a great tool to formally show your commitment to the health and nutrition of the people you serve. The policy can also increase the supply of healthy food in your inventory. You can incorporate a nutrition policy into your organization's mission statement, on your website, and in your donor appeals to focus on not just providing pounds of food to those in need but high quality, nutritious food to promote health.

The MAZON report released in 2018 documented the degree to which food banks have implemented nutrition policies. Almost two hundred food banks completed the survey, and the results showed the following:

- More than half of food banks have informal nutrition guidelines, and one-third have formal nutrition policies; 85 percent of these food banks report that this has not negatively impacted annual donations or pounds.
- One out of seven food banks have formally banned some items, such as soda and candy, as part of their nutrition policy.

Rather than a yes/no scenario (you either take all donations or say no to donations), think of nutrition standards and policies as an opportunity to build a closer relationship with your food donors.

I've included resources for creating a nutrition policy in the resource section at the end of this chapter. You don't have to start from scratch. The MAZON report found that nearly 40 percent of food banks with nutrition policies and guidelines are unsure how to handle unwanted food and beverage donations. More than half of food banks have begun educating local food and beverage donors about the need for more nutritious donations, yet only one-fifth have approached national donors.

Rather than a yes/no scenario (you either take all donations or say no to donations), think of nutrition standards and policies as an opportunity to build a closer relationship with your food donors. You can have conversations about the types of food they donate and the types of food that would be most beneficial to your food bank or pantry and the people you serve. Yes, food donors may be looking for a tax break from their donated product, but they want to be strong community partners too.

Jason Jakubowski, president and CEO of Foodshare, describes the importance of relationships when developing a nutrition policy: "When we developed our nutrition policy here at Foodshare, we deliberately made it an inclusive process. We created a dynamic dialogue between our food donors, our staff, and ultimately our board members. The process itself probably took longer, but by the time it was fully vetted, there was no dissension and our board approved it unanimously." Food banks and food pantries often view their relationship with food donors as a one-way street. The donor provides food, and we are grateful for whatever we can get. We want to shift the dynamic to a relationship that is mutually beneficial.

The Capital Area Food Bank in Washington, DC, has long been an advocate for health and nutrition, and they adopted a strong food policy that limits donations with high sugar content from retailers. Their experience is an example of why nutrition policies can be beneficial and how to build relationships with food donors to provide healthier food. The food bank had been receiving large quantities of sheet cakes but did not want to distribute so many to their network, so they were stockpiling them in their warehouse cooler. Finally, Nancy Roman, the director at the time, had a conversation with the grocery store to ask why they were donating so many cakes. The grocery store manager had no idea that they were making so many extra cakes because the donations were leaving the store and going to the food bank. Out of sight, out of mind. He notified his staff to reduce the amount of cake they made, and the food bank did not have to dispose of unwanted cake. The retail store partnered with the food bank and became a champion to help support their nutrition work.

Another great opportunity for food banks that are committed to health and nutrition is to become a partner with Partnership for a Healthier America (PHA), a national organization founded by former first lady Michelle Obama as part of her Let's Move campaign to prevent childhood obesity and led by Nancy Roman, who has strong food banking experience. By partnering with PHA, food banks commit to using a nutrition ranking system to determine the nutritional quality of their food, increasing the supply and distribution of healthy food, decreasing the supply of less healthy food, and providing incentives for food pantries to promote healthy food.

Healthy Donations to Food Pantries

A couple of years ago I was at a food pantry and a nice couple pulled into the parking lot to deliver donations. They opened the back of their truck and unloaded several cases of ramen noodle containers. They said they were on sale. I know their hearts were in the right place, but ramen noodles are one of the easiest and cheapest items to get when you're on a tight budget, and they are chock-full of sodium.

Just as food banks receive unhealthy donations from retailers, food pantries face similar challenges with local food drives from churches, scout groups, schools, and local businesses. People who donate food to pantries want to be helpful. They will often appreciate direction for what would be most beneficial to the organization. I suggest to food pantry staff that they let donors know they are concerned about the health and well-being of their clients and provide a list of healthy items they need most. This may take time to sink in and to change the mindset of donors who have been donating canned soup for years, but change can happen. We have created a healthy food donation list and other materials to describe the importance of promoting healthy food in a pantry setting, and I've included a link to our website in the resource list. Rather than being offended, I believe most donors want their donation to be useful for the pantry. It helps to have strong leadership to reinforce these messages.

Another suggestion for food pantries is to ask donors for a specific food item that is difficult to get from the food bank and that you know is in demand by your guests. For example, run a cereal drive, and let donors know you prefer cereal with less than six grams of sugar. You can also run a diaper drive to help families with young children, or a toilet paper drive. It will be easier for your food pantry staff and volunteers to sort through the donations when you are receiving similar items rather than hundreds of bags of totally miscellaneous food items that you may or may not want for your food pantry.

You can also run a diaper drive to help families with young children, or a toilet paper drive.

Some food pantries are not currently equipped to handle perishable items because they lack refrigeration or storage areas for fresh produce, dairy, and meat. Thankfully, this is changing. Many food banks are providing equipment grants to food pantries to purchase refrigerators and shelves. Some large name retailers such as Walmart and Coca-Cola replace their refrigerators in retail stores frequently and may be willing to donate their used equipment. It is worth asking. Food banks are also partnering with retail grocery stores and gaining access to more donated perishable food items and are working with food pantries to receive more perishable food.

You may think that you cannot offer fresh produce or other perishables in your pantry. I would encourage you to reconsider. In the last chapter on offering client choice, I provided some recommendations for displaying food for guests to choose. Here are a few additional considerations you will need to make when offering perishables:

- You will need refrigerators to store produce. We recommend glass-front refrigerators so guests can see what is inside.
- You will need shelving and display bins specifically for produce. A lot of produce can be displayed beautifully with limited or no refrigeration.
- You will want to pick up perishables the day before or the day of your distributions.
- You might designate volunteers to sort through and display produce. Ask if volunteers have a background in gardening. This isn't the most glamorous job, but it is important.
- You will have more garbage to dispose of from rotten produce, so consider your trash pickup schedule. You might also consider creating a compost.
- You may still want to set limits on how many items guests can choose, such as two per family. But if you have a large amount of perishable items, you may consider allowing guests as many as they like so you don't have as much requiring disposal.

Healthy Choices Made Easier

Many people who visit a food pantry already want to eat healthier, and the most important thing the staff can do is make nutritious food available. Yet all of us could use a little nudge to make better choices. Education is often the go-to answer, but research from the field of psychology shows that information alone is not very successful at helping people change behavior. Instead, it is more effective to change the environment. Think about the example of the hardware store checkout. Even though you came to buy paint, the environment makes it very easy and convenient to buy a candy bar, or even two because they're on sale and they are right next to the register.

The field of behavioral economics illustrates how small changes to our environments can make the healthy choice the easier choice. Most of us don't like to go out of our way to make a decision or a change, so if the default option is the healthy option, people will likely choose it. This is where the idea of "nudges" come into play—subtle cues to help people make healthy choices. Most of us don't like to be told what we *should* do, but if you get a little nudge in the right direction it is more appealing and you're more likely to follow through with a change.

A few examples of healthy nudges include placing fruit by the checkout counter, reducing the cost of the healthy lunch in a cafeteria compared with a higher-fat lunch, and making low-fat milk the default option for kids' meals at a restaurant instead of soda. Feeding America created a Nudges Toolkit to promote healthy food in food pantries. Here are examples of using nudges within a food pantry setting:

- Place fresh fruits and vegetables at the beginning of the pantry distribution or on the display ends of shelves and include signage in multiple languages to promote them.
- Create a convenient "meal kit" by bundling healthy options that are hard to move with more familiar options, such as brown rice with beans and corn. When packaged together, they look more like a meal.
- Provide taste tests for healthy items in addition to a recipe.

The SWAP System: Supporting Wellness at Pantries

After spending a great deal of time in food pantries, and encouraging pantry directors to provide more healthy food, I realized that many of us, including pantry directors and volunteers, could benefit from a tool to help determine what food is actually "healthy." This is how I decided to create the SWAP system, which stands for Supporting Wellness at Pantries. I partnered closely with Marlene Schwartz at the Rudd Center for Food Policy and Obesity and Michelle McCabe from the Council of Churches of Greater Bridgeport to pilot test and revise the system in food pantries.

SWAP is a stoplight nutrition system that ranks food as green (choose often), yellow (choose sometimes), and red (choose rarely) based on the amount of saturated fat, sodium, and sugar in the food. We focus on these three nutrients because they are the ones most associated with chronic disease risk. Based on the most recent Dietary Guidelines for Americans issued by the federal government, SWAP is a simple and intuitive way to determine which food items are healthier than others. We use the stoplight symbol because it is easy to understand even if English is not your first language or if you have low literacy skills.

Looking even further upstream, by identifying and promoting healthy food items in a food bank's inventory, SWAP can also influence food companies and manufacturers to improve the nutritional quality of the food they make and donate to food banks.

The goal of SWAP is to improve the supply and demand for healthy food within food banks and food pantries. The intended audience for SWAP is the end user, the families who shop at pantries and are often struggling with a chronic disease and want to make healthier food choices. But SWAP is also beneficial for food pantry directors and food bank staff members to make healthier decisions when they order food and also for people who donate food to a food pantry. In fact, because SWAP is such an easy tool for ranking food nutritionally, it is useful for anyone interested in making healthy food choices.

Looking even further upstream, by identifying and promoting healthy food items in a food bank's inventory, SWAP can also influence food companies and manufacturers to improve the nutritional quality of the food they make and donate to food banks. Food banks can provide reports of the nutritional quality of donated food to the food donors and companies who produce the food. This is an opportunity to let them know that we are concerned about the nutritional quality of food that is available for food pantry customers. Over time, this can help improve the supply of healthy food that comes into the charitable food system.

I had a pleasant surprise when Anita Shaffer, a senior nutrition manager from Campbell Soup Company, contacted me because she had read about the SWAP system and wanted to see how the food that they sell directly to Feeding America ranked according to SWAP. She said, "I will be making recommendations to my team to modify the mix for a better nutrition profile." This is where real systems change can take place. Yes, we need to provide nutrition education to customers who shop at food pantries, but improving the nutritional quality of the food that is donated to food banks can create large-scale health benefits. In order to improve the charitable food system, we need help with both the supply of and demand for healthy food.

Currently, several food banks are using SWAP to rank their food, and dozens of food pantries around the country are using SWAP with promotional posters and shelf tags. The director of a food bank in Oregon said, "The SWAP system is a food bank dietician's dream!" Lisa Diewald, a program manager at the MacDonald Center for Obesity Prevention and Education at Villanova University, helped to implement the SWAP system in a local food pantry. She commented, "Since our last conversation, we've trained the key volunteers in the pantry on SWAP as well as our 10 peer mentors. They learned quickly and the SWAP food category excel spreadsheet you sent recently has been SO helpful!"

Maria Delis, the nutrition education coordinator/dietitian at a food pantry outside Chicago also found the tool helpful, writing, "Our staff is so bought into this program that we have revised all of our tracking documents to reflect SWAP guidelines, our volunteers who sort are all trained on SWAP, and our executive director is using the program results to solicit grant money for the pantry. In addition, our big school food drive in April has been revised to emphasize SWAP!" This pantry is a great example of the paradigm shift in charitable food. They recently changed their name from the Oak Park River Forest Food Pantry to Beyond Hunger. They are focusing on healthy, nutritious food and much more.

Health Promotion and Trauma-informed Care

In our messaging and training about the SWAP system, we make it clear that "red" food items don't mean "never eat." We all like red foods occasionally, but we describe them as treats and items you should choose rarely. We highlight the importance of providing client choice and allowing guests to choose their food with dignity. The red label should not be designed to shame or blame people for their food choices.

In chapter 4, I discussed the importance of recognizing how trauma impacts people who are food insecure and how food banks and food pantries should pay attention to how we design and operate our programs to reduce harm and potential trauma. You may be thinking, how does this relate to nutrition and the SWAP system? Bear with me, it comes together.

When you have a crappy day or are feeling low, what type of food do you crave? When you have a great day and have something to celebrate, what food do you seek? There is an important time and place for red foods, the "choose rarely" foods. As much as we want to emphasize healthy, nutritious food within food pantry settings, we can also create space for treats too. And we can do it in a way that promotes the overall well-being of food pantry guests. Enjoying an occasional dessert, feeling seen and appreciated by food pantry staff and volunteers, will help fill the soul.

Having a section of your pantry that has reasonable-sized desserts can be appealing. Unfortunately, many food banks and food pantries are receiving donations from retail grocery stores with oversized cakes, pies, and cookie trays designed for a company outing, not a family of three. And because they are perishable, food pantries have a need to distribute or dispose of these items.

Are there opportunities to cut up a sheet cake and invite guests to have a slice of cake after they shop and to socialize with others at the pantry? Similar to the Capital Area Food Bank example, if you routinely receive bulk desserts, this may be an opportunity to talk with your grocery store to see why they are producing so many desserts that they need to donate them. Can the grocery store repackage bulk donations into smaller portions that are appropriate for a family?

Unfortunately, many food banks and food pantries are receiving donations from retail grocery stores with oversized cakes, pies, and cookie trays designed for a company outing, not a family of three.

Household Items

In addition to focusing on the nutritional quality of food, another innovative step that many food pantries take is to stock shelves with non-food items. It is important to recognize that if people are in need of food, they also need help with household products such as toilet paper, cleaning supplies, diapers, laundry detergent, feminine products, and so on. These are often expensive items, and you can't use SNAP dollars to purchase them because SNAP can only be used to purchase food.

These items are not only necessary but help us feel human. Food banks and food pantries can think about ways to solicit donations for these nonfood items.

It can be enlightening for local donors to recognize how hunger can impact a household. People who cannot afford food also cannot afford other basic necessities. This can help build empathy. But many food pantries are just that—pantries filled with food. There is no reason you cannot offer many additional items to help families make ends meet.

Healthy Pantry Programs

Many food banks have designated nutrition staff who provide nutrition education and provide resources to promote healthy food. Some food banks are hiring researchers and nutritionists to help advance their work in health and nutrition. If you are a student in nutrition or public health, consider a community nutrition job or internship at a food bank. We need your expertise.

The VT Fresh program doesn't just increase the supply of healthy produce, they focus on making sure the display of produce is beautiful to help increase the demand as well.

An early champion in the work of bringing more produce into food pantries is the Vermont Foodbank's VT Fresh program. If they can promote beautiful, healthy, fresh produce in a northern state like Vermont that has a very short growing season, certainly we can add more produce to our local food pantries. The VT Fresh program provides small grants to food pantries to increase food pantry capacity to stock and promote fruits and vegetables. In 2018, they reported a 230 percent average increase in pounds of produce distributed by participating food pantries. As part of the SNAP-Ed program, VT Fresh offers cooking demonstrations and taste tests so guests can sample the food that is available at the pantries. They conducted pre–post tests to measure changes and found impressive results. Among over two hundred people who participated in the direct nutrition education, 25 percent reported an increase in daily vegetable consumption and 19 percent said they were eating more fruits on a daily basis.

The VT Fresh program doesn't just increase the supply of healthy produce, they focus on making sure the display of produce is beautiful to help increase the demand as well. Michelle Wallace, the director of VT Fresh, describes how "the program has directly impacted the organization's systems and ability to procure, display, sort and promote fresh foods. The program has also impacted the organizational culture of each of these organizations towards valuing and prioritizing fresh produce." The VT Fresh program was promoting healthy nudges before nudges became popular.

The Capital Area Food Bank has a wellness program to identify nutritious food and recipes for their member food pantries to promote healthy food with food available from the food bank. The Greater Boston Food Bank has a team of registered dietitians who provide nutrition education through newsletters, recipes, educational programs, and resources. Researchers at the University of Minnesota have developed healthy pantry initiatives and studied the impact on food supply and choices made by guests. I could probably write an entire book just on promoting healthy food in food banks and pantries, but I'm trying to provide the highlights in one chapter. Suffice it to say that interest in this work is growing rapidly, and there are many examples of innovative healthy pantry programs nationwide.

In 2019, Healthy Eating Research (HER), a national program of the Robert Wood Johnson Foundation, convened an expert panel of nutrition professionals and food bank staff members to develop nutrition guidelines for the charitable food system. I was proud to serve on the panel, and we used the SWAP guidelines as a foundational reference point for creating the new guidelines. In 2020, Feeding America adopted the HER guidelines and will encourage food banks to rank food nutritionally using the new guidelines. This is a clear example of reinventing the role of food banks! It represents a milestone in our efforts to promote healthy food within food banks and food pantries.

Good nutrition at food pantries is largely a health issue, but it is also a matter of social justice. It is about leveling the playing field so people who are food insecure are not further encumbered by health problems linked to poor diet. We should all be able to eat healthy food, regardless of income or zip code.

Action Steps

- Take a good look at the types of food that are offered in your food bank or food pantry. Discuss the connection between hunger and health with your staff and volunteers, provide data outlined in this chapter, and describe why it is hard to access healthy, affordable food on a limited budget.
- Consider using a nutrition ranking system like SWAP to determine the nutritional quality of the food you provide so you can increase the supply and demand of healthy food. I'm happy to get you started.
- Use "nudges" to make the healthy choice the easier choice at your food pantry. Think like a marketer to "sell" the healthier options with signs, displays, and promotions.
- Ask food donors for specific healthy items that are hard to get at the food bank. You can use a healthy food donation list.
- Partner with health care providers such as clinics or hospitals to screen patients for food insecurity and chronic diseases and help link them to healthy food pantries.

- Implement a nutrition policy at your food bank or food pantry to show your commitment to health and wellness.
- Partner with nutrition and dietetic professionals to provide recipes, classes, and workshops on nutrition.

What step will you take toward promoting healthy food?

Resources

Feldman, Marla, and Marlene B. Schwartz. "A Tipping Point: Leveraging Opportunities to Improve the Nutritional Quality of Food Bank Inventory." MAZON (March 2018). https://mazon.org/assets/download-files/MAZON -TippingPointReport-FINAL.pdf.

Healthy Eating Research. "Nutrition Guidelines for the Charitable Food System." March 2020. https://healthyeatingresearch.org/wp-content/uploads/2020/02 /her-food-bank_FINAL.pdf.

Hunger + Health/Feeding America. https://hungerandhealth.feedingamerica.org/.

Hunger + Health/Feeding America. "The Power of Nudges: Making the Healthy Choice the Easy Choice in Food Pantries." https://hungerandhealth.feeding america.org/resource/the-power-of-nudges-making-the-healthy-choice-the -easy-choice-in-food-pantries/.

Martin, Katie, Michele Wolff, Kate Callahan, and Marlene Schwartz. "Supporting Wellness at Pantries: Development of a Nutrition Stoplight System for Food Banks and Food Pantries." *Journal of the Academy of Nutrition and Dietetics* 119, no. 4 (2018): 553–558. https://doi.org/10.1016/j.jand.2018.03.003.

Partnership for a Healthier America. https://www.ahealthieramerica.org/.

Pollan, Michael. *The Omnivore's Dilemma: A Natural History of Four Meals.* New York: Penguin Press, 2006.

Schwartz, Marlene B., and Hilary K. Seligman. "The Unrealized Health-Promoting Potential of a National Network of Food Pantries." *Journal of Hunger & Environmental Nutrition* 14, no. 1–2 (2019): 1–3. https://doi.org/10.1080 /19320248.2019.1569819.

Vermont Foodbank. "VT Fresh." https://www.vtfoodbank.org/nurture-people /vt-fresh.

CHAPTER 7
Connection to Community Services

In the last few chapters, we've talked about designing food pantries to promote dignity and health. But let's take a step back and think about why individuals come to the food pantry in the first place. Yes, they are coming for food and will be grateful to receive it. We can see the immediate need firsthand as people wait in line at food pantries. But food is just the tip of the iceberg and often one of the easier challenges to solve. Larger and more complicated needs lie below the surface.

The primary role of food banks and food pantries, from their beginnings forty years ago to today, is to distribute food. That is because we often view the problem of hunger as simply a lack of food, and we describe our efforts largely in terms of how many pounds of food we have distributed to solve the problem. Even when that food is nutritious and provided with dignity, it is addressing the short-term problem. By focusing only on food, we miss the opportunity to help people address other challenges in their lives that contribute to their food insecurity. We can design food pantries as a platform to offer wraparound services and a space for community engagement.

When we recognize that the underlying causes of hunger are largely rooted in poverty and systemic inequalities, then our responses become more holistic. By connecting families who are food insecure to available community services, we can begin to address their situation beyond food. This is a shift from the transaction of providing food toward relational work that helps clients build stability and self-sufficiency. The food can serve as the literal and figurative "carrot," the reason why people come to the pantry, but it can also lead to other, more fundamental kinds of help.

Our Mission

It wasn't long ago that the idea of providing resources beyond food, such as SNAP outreach, was seen as mission creep, or veering away from the fundamental role of food banks and food pantries. You may still hear these concerns from some staff, volunteers, or board members. If the mission of a food bank or pantry is to "feed the hungry," then staff may question the idea of committing limited resources to anything but collecting and distributing food. But isn't our mission to do more than simply provide food? I believe so.

Many long-time directors never dreamed that they would be running a food bank or pantry for decades. They are increasingly recognizing that food alone is not eliminating the need for food, and they are looking for new ways to serve the people who come to their programs for help. Many food banks and pantries are developing innovative approaches to provide additional amenities, trainings, and programs. If we are serious about tackling hunger, connecting people to additional services should be viewed as directly in line with our mission.

Nick Saul describes this broader role of a food pantry in his compelling and thought-provoking book *The Stop*. He says, "Instead of simply 'feeding the need' by handing out food—a one-off transaction—there is incredible potential here at The Stop to engage with the people of this neighborhood to take charge of their own lives. To provide support as they articulate and work toward their own dreams for the future." If we view our customers as vital and valuable members of our community, we know that food is just one aspect of their well-being.

It can be helpful to ask yourself: are we in the business of feeding people, or helping to solve the problem of hunger? Kristen Miale, president of the Good Shepherd Food Bank in Maine, describes the difference between "going deep with a few" strategies versus "going narrow with many." This shift in thinking will move us from an emergency response with a handout to empowering people with a hand up. Remember, this doesn't have to be an either/or scenario. You can continue to provide short-term food supplies to many people in your distribution line, AND you can also begin to offer deeper connections and one-on-one support with people who are interested and ready for additional help.

You can continue to provide short-term food supplies to many people in your distribution line, AND you can also begin to offer deeper connections and one-on-one support with people who are interested and ready for additional help.

This paradigm shift is a key step in how we can reinvent the way we provide charitable food in America. The shift will rely on the firm belief that it takes more than food to end hunger. Like many tools we are discussing throughout this book, please don't view this approach as all or nothing. I describe various steps you can take to provide referrals and to connect your guests with other antihunger and antipoverty programs and services in your community.

In this chapter, we focus on working at the individual level to help increase a family's financial resources, human capital, and social capital so they can access and afford enough food. I describe various ways to address the root causes of hunger by collaborating with community programs and services to build collective impact. I provide information about an evidence-based program called More Than Food, which is a strength-based and nonjudgmental approach to help people set and reach goals in their lives. Hopefully you will find some tools that you'd like to try.

Needs beyond Food

Studies show that families have to make really difficult trade-off decisions when they are food insecure. The national Hunger in America study from 2014 found that the majority of households who use the charitable food system had to choose between paying for food and paying for utilities (69 percent), transportation (67 percent), medical care (66 percent), housing (57 percent), or education (31 percent) at some point in the past twelve months. During spring 2020 of the COVID-19 pandemic, I conducted brief surveys with families coming to pick up food at a drive-through distribution program. Because of the economic impact, 69 percent of households said they had to choose between paying for food and paying other bills during the past month. Food is one basic need, but there are many other pressing and competing priorities that families face on a monthly basis.

Food pantries can serve as ideal settings to help address these other basic needs. The 2014 Hunger in America study found that among the national network of food pantries and meal programs, about one-third (35 percent) connect individuals and families with nonfood programs or services. These connections help guests address the other economic and social hardships they may face, in addition to short-term food supplies. Among the food pantries and meal programs that offer these additional services,

- 40 percent help clients enroll in SNAP;
- 35 percent help families connect with other benefits and nonfood needs; and
- 30 percent help clients enroll in Medicaid.

Because this was the last national study that was conducted through the Feeding America network of food pantries, these numbers have likely increased over the past several years. But you can also see that there is a lot of room for growth. Over half of hunger relief organizations are not providing outreach or services beyond food. We can do better. We can aim higher.

Connection to Community Services

Offering services beyond food in a food pantry setting can take several different approaches. Just like the examples of providing choice within a food pantry, moving beyond food distribution can be seen along a continuum. The goal is to start where you are comfortable and then move along the continuum to offer more services. There are simple things you can do to get started and then build additional resources over time. Consider the following examples of connecting clients to community services, from basic to advanced:

- Hang flyers about available community programs and services on a bulletin board.
- Have a volunteer who is knowledgeable about local services available to hand out flyers or brochures.
- Have a bulletin board where guests can post services needed or skills available, such as child care, transportation, or jobs. This can be an opportunity for guests, volunteers, and staff to match and trade available skills with needed services.
- Invite health and social service providers to come to your pantry to describe their services and help enroll clients in their programs.
- Offer classes and workshops, such as computer skills or English as a second language, on-site at the pantry.
- Train a coach to provide case management services and work one-on-one with individuals to set goals and build food security.

When we recognize that lack of food is just one factor affecting a household, it makes sense to provide information about other community programs and services that will help increase food security. For example, you can set up an area in your pantry as a resource center with information about community organizations that provide child care, utility assistance, GED classes, job training programs, nutrition education, voter registration, housing assistance, legal assistance, SNAP enrollment, and other services.

Many social service agencies or United Way programs have a guide of local community resources. You'll want to start here and not re-create the wheel. Find out what other programs and services already exist for your guests to access. Researching these services can be a great project for a student intern or regular volunteer. Once these resources are identified, the intern or volunteer can call various organizations and talk with service providers to learn more about their programs, hours of operation, eligibility criteria, and how best to refer people from the food pantry to enroll in available programs.

Ideally, a staff member or volunteer would meet with representatives from local agencies so when a client is interested, the volunteer or staff member can provide a "warm" referral because that individual has firsthand knowledge about the local resources rather than simply a brochure. Providing referrals is a good first step, but it's even more beneficial if there is at least one follow-up conversation to see if the client took advantage of the referral or if the client had barriers. We call this *relational work* because it involves getting to know individuals who come to your pantry, building relationships, and following up with them.

Collective Impact

Connecting people to community services does not mean that your pantry has to be an expert on all of these issues or that you need to

Rather than working in silos, we will have a greater impact in our communities when antihunger organizations partner with other social service organizations for a collective approach.

actually provide these services within your pantry. But it is important to have a good understanding of what community agencies, services, and programs exist in your local area that will benefit your guests. Addressing root causes of hunger is a big job, and we can't do it alone. Find ways to partner and collaborate with others who are doing good antipoverty work in your community to build collective impact. Rather than working in silos, we will have a greater impact in our communities when antihunger organizations partner with other social service organizations for a collective approach. We don't have to duplicate services—this is an opportunity to partner with existing community programs and provide wraparound services.

Once you start to provide information about community programs and connect clients to these services, you will have a better understanding of the common challenges and needs that exist for your clientele. In a rural community, transportation may be a barrier. In an urban area, it may be utility assistance. A next step beyond referrals is to design a one-stop-shopping experience to make it convenient for your guests to receive assistance. For example, the Kelly Hunger Relief Center in El Paso, Texas, hosts resource fairs where they invite representatives from several community programs to come to the pantry to provide information on-site and to enroll people in their programs. This is a win-win situation because the food pantry helps connect their guests to valuable services and the social service programs have a convenient location for recruitment.

One of the barriers that you may encounter when you first provide information about community programs is that guests may seem disinterested and focused only on getting food. It may take time to shift the focus of your pantry from food distribution to food and resources to one-stop shopping. Relationships are critical here. It helps if you have a staff or volunteer who is a familiar face, preferably from the community and possibly a guest of the pantry, who can encourage food pantry guests to check out additional services and help enroll them into programs. In chapter 4 I mentioned the benefit of having a greeter at the pantry who welcomes people and provides a friendly face. They should wear a name tag. This person can also introduce guests to the new resource center and help recruit people to check out additional programs.

It may take time to shift the focus of your pantry from food distribution to food and resources to one-stop shopping.

Duplication of Services

There is a common misperception about social services for people in poverty. Many people believe that if you have a low income, then you are automatically assigned to a case manager and are familiar with available social service programs. Typically, the concern about providing referrals and case management within a food pantry setting is that this will duplicate efforts that are already being provided by other social service organizations. Sadly, this is not the reality.

Living in poverty is isolating, and it is challenging to try to navigate the complex bureaucracy of getting help. Social service programs often involve a great deal of red tape and have tremendous caseloads, so even if an individual is assigned to a caseworker, that assignment is specific to participation in one program. One of the coaches that is trained in the More Than Food program in Rhode Island said, "People assume if you receive SNAP that you receive all the other programs. That's not the case." She said she wanted to be part of the Fresh Start program that offers case management because, "I want to be part of a program that I wish someone had provided for my parents."

Recognizing that people have needs beyond food, when I conducted surveys in spring 2020 during COVID-19 at Foodshare's food distribution site, I asked people, "If there were a program where you could talk with a coach over the phone to help with applying for services, budgeting money, and other support, would you be interested in talking with a coach about goals?" The majority of people (over 55 percent) said they would be interested. Yes, people are in need of food, and they are also looking for additional support and connection. One woman said, "I want to work on my credit so I'll be able to afford to get a house and be able to pay my mortgage and save money as well." Another guest said, "It would help to talk to a coach to determine what money to put where for essential bills."

More Than Food

Katy Bunder, the CEO of Food Finders food bank in Lafayette, Indiana, was searching for a new space to provide more wraparound services at their food bank. She looked at nineteen different locations. She knew it had to be on the bus line to be convenient for the people they were serving. She had read articles about Freshplace in Hartford, Connecticut, and wanted to create a similar holistic food pantry model. When I went to visit, I was anticipating a typical food bank with a large industrial warehouse building and a large parking lot. But that's not what I found. Their office doesn't look like much from the street. In fact, I passed right by it and had to drive around the block. They do have a warehouse building, but it is located a few blocks away. Their smaller office is in a residential neighborhood close to a bus line and serves as their food resource center where they connect people to other human services. When people come to the pantry, they meet with a case manager who helps inform them of additional programs that can help beyond food. Food Finders is exploring ways to provide more in-depth case management services and following clients over time.

If you are ready to dig deeper in this area, and go beyond referrals, you can designate a coach to work with food pantry guests and provide one-on-one case management with follow-ups. More Than Food is a holistic approach to addressing the root causes of food insecurity, helping individuals reach goals so they will not need to rely on food pantries over the long-term. It is an example of reinventing the focus of a food pantry from emergency to empowerment.

More Than Food is a holistic approach to addressing the root causes of food insecurity, helping individuals reach goals so they will not need to rely on food pantries over the long-term.

More Than Food is a strength-based program that meets people where they are (not just geographically, but emotionally). The focus is nonjudgmental and recognizes that everyone has strengths and dreams for their lives, even if they are in a tough situation at the moment. For the More Than Food framework, we typically call people who participate "members" rather than clients.

The concept of More Than Food started with the Freshplace program in Hartford, Connecticut, and we have replicated the More Than Food program in several food pantries in diverse communities in Greater Hartford, Rhode Island, and El Paso, Texas. My colleagues and I have conducted rigorous evaluations of the program over several years, and we find significant improvements in food security, self-sufficiency, self-efficacy, and diet quality among people who participate. Pantries that offer More Than Food provide client choice and a welcoming environment. But at the heart of offering More Than Food, and the reason I believe we continue to find significant results from members who participate, is individualized coaching. I'll describe the training and the process we use for coaches to work with members. But first, I want to explain the theory we use that guides this work.

Change Doesn't Happen Overnight

Building long-term food security means helping people make changes in their life. This can be joining a job training program, going back to school, or enrolling in a nutrition education class. But most human beings don't like change. We like the comfort of the status quo. So how do we motivate people to make a change in their life? The More Than Food program is rooted in a theory called Stages of Change, which recognizes that behavior change happens in phases, not all at once. Stages of Change has been used widely with addictions, helping people to quit smoking or abusing drugs and alcohol. Think about it: if someone is not considering quitting smoking, if you were to provide them with the best program for smoking cessation, it wouldn't be effective because the person is not ready to try it.

The More Than Food program is rooted in a theory called Stages of Change, which recognizes that behavior change happens in phases, not all at once.

Unfortunately, too often we design and introduce programs that assume everyone is ready to make a change in their life. While well intentioned, we often become discouraged and frustrated when people don't take advantage of our programs, for example, when no one shows up for a budgeting class. I have heard from several food pantry directors who tried a new program, but when people did not take advantage of it, they were reluctant to try another program and focused instead on just providing food.

It can be more effective if a coach has already built a relationship with a member and they have talked about a goal of saving more money.

Having discussions about wanting to save, getting ready, making a plan to save, and then introducing a budgeting class is likely to be more effective.

Providing case management with coaching helps people make positive changes to improve their life situation. For example, a food pantry member may say that they want to complete their GED so they can get a better job. A typical response is to provide a referral for GED classes and expect the person to enroll. All too often we are quick to recognize a goal and move directly to a referral. We hope that since the person stated they want to complete their GED, that providing the appropriate information about the class will be sufficient for follow-up.

But here's the thing. Behavior change is hard, and we need time to prepare for it. Think back to any New Year's resolution you've made and you'll appreciate this. First, we have to recognize an area in our lives that we want to change, decide that we are committed to making a change, start making plans to change, then take baby steps to do things differently, and maintain the change over time. The Stages of Change model is built around the various stages of readiness a person goes through in order to change behavior and make it stick: precontemplation (not even thinking about a change), contemplation, preparation, action, and maintenance. We use this theory to help identify how ready a member is to make a change and then to provide information and motivation based on their stage of readiness.

To return to the earlier example, if someone is thinking about completing their GED, but they haven't made any plans yet, it probably won't be helpful to go online and look at the registration for classes. This may seem intimidating and the member may not sign up. Instead, the coach should determine how important this goal is and how committed the person is to making a change. If the member seems motivated to start the class, the coach may discuss potential barriers and create small steps to prepare for meeting this goal. While this process takes longer than simply handing out a brochure for the GED class, the change is more likely to happen and be sustainable.

It's possible that in order to enroll in the class the member first needs to line up child care for her kids, she may need to save money for the registration fee or to figure out the bus schedule to make sure she can attend the classes after work. A coach can help navigate these additional steps to make sure the referral for GED classes is actually successful. Coaching is also about compassionately holding people accountable for changes they want to make in their lives. Coaches build relationships with members to understand their goals and challenges and to guide them to take the next step. Once an individual is able to accomplish one small goal, they build their confidence, or self-efficacy, in their ability to tackle another goal. Achieving one goal helps build sustainable change over time because when a new challenge arises, as it likely will, the member can lean on their past experience. They will feel more confident in the future to address a new goal.

Achieving one goal helps build sustainable change over time because when a new challenge arises, as it likely will, the member can lean on their past experience.

Coaching Isn't for Everyone

But to be clear, not everyone is interested in or ready for individualized attention and working with a coach at a food pantry. The program isn't a great fit for everyone. By using Stages of Change, you can help identify how ready and motivated a person is to make changes in their life. If a person is in crisis mode, focused on getting enough food to last the next few days, trying to keep their lights on this month, and generally in the precontemplation phase, they are not a great fit for a coaching program. You want to recruit people who talk about wanting more for their kids, who are ready to go back to school, who are looking for a better job. Recruit people who are contemplating or planning to make a change in their life. These are good candidates for this type of holistic approach.

It's helpful to remember that if you offer coaching in a food pantry setting, you won't be offering case management for everyone who attends your pantry. You can continue to provide your traditional food services for your full clientele and then select a smaller group of people who are ready to be part of the more intensive coaching program. For the More Than Food program, we recommend that a pantry have one full-time staff member who oversees the overall pantry program and then a coach who can work part-time, ideally in a paid rather than volunteer position. It is best if the coach can meet with members in a private area during a separate time than the regular food pantry distribution.

While we use Stages of Change to help determine how ready an individual is to make a change, we can also apply the theory to organizations.

While we use Stages of Change to help determine how ready an individual is to make a change, we can also apply the theory to organizations. When I talk with food pantry directors about incorporating client choice or promoting healthy food or offering More Than Food, I try to gauge what stage of readiness they are in and then provide information to help them move to the next stage. This is really about meeting people and organizations where they are and encouraging them to take one step toward the next level of action or programming.

Motivational Interviewing

In our More Than Food program, we provide standardized training for coaches to help individuals identify areas in their life that are holding them back from being food secure and help them set up to three initial goals for becoming more food secure and financially stable. The program is designed to recruit members who seem ready for change and to provide one-on-one coaching over six to nine months. Coaches typically meet with members twice per month for three months, then once per month for an additional three to six months. We have a training manual, standardized program forms, and evaluation tools to measure changes. During COVID-19, we plan to offer virtual coaching in lieu of face-to-face meetings.

We provide training for coaches to offer case management using Motivational Interviewing (or MI for short), which is often used within social work programs. Motivational Interviewing is designed to increase a person's commitment to a specific goal by discussing the person's own reasons for change. This is not a cookie-cutter, one-size-fits-all approach but is tailored to the individual situation of each person's life. Using MI techniques, coaches build relationships with members and help boost their self-efficacy to reach their goals. Rather than expecting someone to make a long-term plan or to drastically change their behavior, we focus on and celebrate small steps.

The coaches use open-ended questions to help members identify areas in their life that they want to improve. Motivational Interviewing recognizes that making a change requires importance, commitment, and confidence. The coach can help identify how important the goal is and how committed and confident the member is to work toward this goal. For example, it may be very important for a person to pay the rent so they don't get evicted, but they may lack confidence in their ability to save extra money. The coach can help build their motivation and readiness to start a budgeting class to help pay the rent.

Coaches work one-on-one with individuals to connect them with community resources and programs that will build their self-sufficiency, such as job training, education, skill building, and nutrition education. The Fresh Start program at the Kelly Center for Hunger Relief in El

Paso, Texas, has been offering More Than Food since 2017, and they have hosted three graduation ceremonies to celebrate the accomplishments of members who have completed the nine-month program.

A recent graduate at the Fresh Start program in El Paso explained, "Joining helped me to deal with my depression and anxiety. I got to know other members and we became friends. My three goals were finding an apartment, finding a job, and my US citizenship. So little by little, I came to the program and talked to them about my goals. They would encourage me, and I felt more confident. The first thing that I got was my job, then my citizenship. Then, after time, I found an apartment."

More Than Food can boost financial resources by helping members enroll in SNAP or in budgeting classes. Members can increase their human capital by enrolling in job training programs and education programs to build skills and knowledge. The program can also raise social capital because members build networks with their coach and other members in the program who support one another toward similar goals. Offering More Than Food helps create a community space, where people come not just for food but for connection, support, and encouragement.

A coach in Rhode Island described the progress of a member who was graduating from the program: "Overall, crises decreased; increased stability, income, and mental health. Still hopes to advance in career or jobs. Has more skills to make changes independently."

A Focus on Strengths

When I was a kid, about once a year *The Wizard of Oz* would be broadcast on TV. These were before the days of instant streaming and hundreds of cable channels available 24/7, so getting a chance to see the movie was a special occasion. I have always been captivated with the story. I love the creative genius of shifting from Dorothy's black and white world in Kansas to the breathtaking panorama of Technicolor sights when Dorothy opens the door into Oz. I enjoy the quirky characters who befriend Dorothy to help her with her goal of getting back to Kansas.

Each of the characters is searching for something they deem lacking in themselves. For Dorothy it is a way to get back home, for the Scarecrow it is brains, the Lion seeks courage, and the Tinman seeks a heart. The moral of the story, of course, is that they had these characteristics inside them all along. Through their adventures in Oz, they tackled their insecurities and built their confidence that they could solve their own problems. They saw the best in each other. All Dorothy had to do was click her heels to get back home.

The role of a coach in the More Than Food program is to recognize the innate strengths in the people they are coaching and help them understand and leverage their own capabilities.

How often do we search outside ourselves for some answer to our problems, only to realize that we hold the solution? The role of a coach in the More Than Food program is to recognize the innate strengths in the people they are coaching and help them understand and leverage their own capabilities. Coaches support members to identify challenges that are holding them back and to build their capacity to help themselves.

Measurement of Impact

One of the most important aspects of More Than Food is that we collect data to track the effectiveness of the program and the impact that it has on people's lives. Very little research of this kind had been conducted previously. Over the past decade, we have learned a lot about the program, what works and doesn't work so well. We continue to iterate and revise as we go. We have created new program materials and continue to evaluate pantries that offer More Than Food. We have standardized case files, survey tools, and exit forms to measure the program and how it helps people. We monitor the data to learn what works and how we can improve services. I provide information on these materials in the resource list. If you're interested, I am happy to get you started.

Coaches are trained to collect informed consent from members and then to conduct surveys when members start the program, again at four months, and between six and nine months after they complete the program. The main outcomes we measure are food security (using the standard USDA food security module), self-sufficiency (using the Missouri Self-Sufficiency Scale), and self-efficacy and sense of control (using the Lachman–Weaver Scale), and we are now measuring financial well-being (using the Consumer Financial Protection Bureau scale). We also ask questions about household demographics, use of food assistance programs, self-reported health outcomes, and trade-off decisions related to food insecurity.

Our research with various food pantries offering More Than Food all have consistent results showing that people who participate in the program have statistically significant increases in food security, self-sufficiency, and self-efficacy over time. We have published several articles describing the methodology and results of our research, and I have included links in the resource section at the end of the chapter. We have evidence to show the program works, and our resources can be helpful tools for others who are interested in offering the program.

Our research with various food pantries offering More Than Food all have consistent results showing that people who participate in the program have statistically significant increases in food security, self-sufficiency, and self-efficacy over time.

More research is needed to evaluate case management services within food pantries and other strategies to end hunger. Feeding America is investing resources in their Ending Hunger Community of Practice, which now includes almost one hundred food banks around the country. They funded a Household Empowerment Pilot program that is very similar to More Than Food and collaborated with the Greater Cleveland Food Bank, Houston Food Bank, and Feeding the Gulf Coast. The three food banks hired coaches to provide case management with motivational interviewing and to connect clients to financial service organizations such as Neighborhood Trust. I served as an advisor for this project, and I was very impressed with the dedication of the food bank staff and their ability to recruit clients into the program.

On-site Classes and Workshops

Another way to offer services beyond food distribution is to provide classes or workshops at your food pantry. As you provide referrals or individualized coaching in your food pantry, you can identify common areas that would benefit many of your clients. Some examples include computer classes, soft skills such as time management, health promotion, and stress reduction. I would encourage you to get creative and think outside the box. Perhaps there is a loyal volunteer at your pantry who would be interested in offering a class or workshop. You can also partner with local social service providers who offer these types of programs and see if they would be willing to offer them at your location.

Connecting clients to social services and offering coaching is a paradigm shift and will reinvent how we provide charitable food. Research shows that we need to examine the underlying reasons people are in the food pantry line and to look beyond food distribution alone. Because it takes more than food to end hunger. This holistic approach requires multiple community agencies working together for collective impact. As we build the capacity of our network to address root causes of hunger, we will improve the health and well-being of people who use our programs so that, ultimately, they will no longer need us.

Action Steps

- Talk with local service providers and United Way to identify the key programs that are available in your community and find existing community resource guides.
- Set up a resource center at your food pantry to connect clients to these services.
- Identify at least one staff member or volunteer who is knowledgeable about these services (or can become so) and can offer referrals.
- Determine if your food bank or food pantry is ready to offer More Than Food; read the resources listed below to help get started.
- Designate a few key staff people who can receive training on the Stages of Change theory and Motivational Interviewing techniques; hire a coach who can work at least part-time with guests.
- Begin recruiting members to participate in the More Than Food program, meet routinely with a coach over a few months. If feasible, collect data to track outcomes.
- Collaborate with other social service providers and antipoverty programs to provide wraparound services.

Are you contemplating and preparing to make a change? What will help motivate you to take action?

Resources

Cherry, Kendra. "The 6 Stages of Behavior Change: The Transtheoretical or Stages of Change Model." Verywell mind. https://www.verywellmind.com /the-stages-of-change-2794868.

Kania, John, and Mark Kramer. "Collective Impact." *Stanford Social Innovation Review* (Winter 2011). https://ssir.org/articles/entry/collective_impact#.

Martin, Katie, Alisha Redelfs, Rong Wu, Olivia Bogner, and Leah Whigham. "Offering More Than Food: Outcomes and Lessons Learned from a Fresh Start Food Pantry in Texas." *Journal of Hunger and Environmental Nutrition* 14, no. 1–2 (2018): 70–81. https://doi.org/10.1080/19320248.2018.1512925.

Motivational Interviewing Network of Trainers. https://motivationalinterview ing.org/.

Sanderson, Jessica, Katie Martin, Angela Colantonio, and Rong Wu. "An Outcome Evaluation of Food Pantries Implementing the More Than Food Framework." *Journal of Hunger and Environmental Nutrition* (2020). https://doi.org /10.1080/19320248.2020.1748782.

CHAPTER 8
The Vital Role of Volunteers

The growth of food banks and food pantries across the country would not be possible without volunteers. In fact, as the charitable food system was developing and taking shape in the 1980s, President George H. W. Bush's address to encourage volunteerism and doing good in one's own community likely spurred the number of volunteers in newly formed food pantries. Unfortunately, this also fundamentally shifted public opinion of the government's role in providing an adequate safety net, placing more responsibility on nonprofit, charitable organizations to pick up the slack. We'll talk about that more in upcoming chapters, but this chapter focuses on the current landscape of volunteer support.

The entire national charitable food system relies on volunteers. According to the 2014 Hunger in America study, among the network of food pantries and community kitchens, on average, only 49 percent report having paid staff. However, the majority of agencies (62 percent) were faith-based organizations, and among this group, less than one-third (32 percent) had paid staff. Therefore, they rely heavily on volunteer support. Among food pantries in the study, the median number of volunteers each month was eighteen, and together they contributed sixty total hours of volunteer time monthly.

Similarly, food banks rely on the important contribution of volunteers. At Foodshare, in 2018, over 6,100 volunteers provided over 47,000 hours of support, which is the equivalent of twenty-four full-time staff members. To put this in context, we have about fifty-five full-time paid staff members. We quite literally could not do the work that we do without volunteers. So what do all of these volunteers do? In this chapter, I'll describe the various jobs performed by volunteers, the invaluable service they provide to charitable food programs, some unfortunate examples of how volunteers can be well-meaning but may cause harm, and suggestions for ensuring that volunteers are aligned with the mission of the food bank or food pantry.

Various Roles of Volunteers

People who volunteer at food banks and food pantries come from all walks of life: retired individuals, faith-based groups, corporate groups, scout organizations, court-appointed individuals who need to perform community service, and families. It is typically a win-win situation in which volunteers receive a great deal of fulfillment and satisfaction from helping others and charitable food programs receive invaluable assistance that they otherwise could not afford. Regular volunteers, often retirees, work routine shifts at a food bank or pantry several times each month to sort and organize food or to do administrative tasks. They typically have an assigned role and perform the same type of duties each time they come to volunteer, and these reliable volunteers, while unpaid, serve similar roles as part-time staff members. Corporate groups, religious organizations, and school groups often sign up for shifts once or several times a year as part of their culture of giving back to the community. Many individuals volunteer periodically, during the holidays or to perform community service.

The vast majority of work conducted by volunteers is food related and involves the physical moving and handling of food, for example,

- Behind the scenes work—sorting, organizing, and shelving food; picking up food from retail stores; and packaging food for distribution; and
- On the front lines—helping during food distributions to check people in to a food pantry and restocking shelves. For traditional food pantries this means helping to prepare and hand out prepacked bags of food, and in client choice pantries this means serving as a co-shopper to assist guests as they choose their food.

Other nonfood related activities can be just as important and involve volunteers sharing their talents and professional expertise in a more directed fashion, for example,

- Administrative help—bookkeeping, answering phones, preparing communication materials;
- Programs and classes—providing nutrition education or budgeting classes, offering referrals to connect clients to community resources;
- Special events—coordinating, staffing, sending invitations, promoting on social media;
- Fundraising—helping with grant writing; being an ambassador to recruit new donors; and
- Leadership—serving on boards of directors, advisory groups, or committees.

There are many standard roles that volunteers serve within charitable food programs, and I would encourage staff members to get creative and think outside the box for new roles. Are there projects or is there work to be done that you don't have staff capacity for but which could be performed by a volunteer? The Mount Kisco Interfaith Food Pantry in New York describes how their food pantry is administered by "the Board and a part-time Director of Operations and Programs, with the invaluable assistance of hundreds of regular volunteers. The Board is organized around working committees: Management, Finance, Operations, Governance, Grants, and Development. Our nearly-all-volunteer model means that there are many ways that volunteers can apply their skills to the Pantry's mission."

Volunteers are the lifeblood of food banks and food pantries and provide critical programming support. However, unintended consequences can occur if there are flaws in how we structure our services to accommodate volunteers or in the ways that volunteers interact with food pantry guests.

The Interests of Volunteers and Guests— Who Are We Serving?

In our important efforts to provide charitable food, we need to look closely at our work and ask some hard questions. Are we providing food and services in ways that benefit our volunteers and donors or our neighbors who don't have enough to eat? Are we serving the interests of volunteers and donors over the needs of our community? This sounds obvious, but many decisions and ways of operating programs are based on the convenience and for the benefit of volunteers.

Are we serving the interests of volunteers and donors over the needs of our community?

It is important to do a gut check every once in a while, to take stock of how, when, and where our food banks and food pantries operate. When you think about the days and hours of operation and how food is collected and distributed—are these operations based on what is most convenient for volunteers? Or do we focus our programs on what is most needed and convenient for our guests, paying attention to what is conducive for working families?

As we discussed with choice, prepacking and distributing food to people in line creates clear roles and jobs for volunteers but is not ideal for our guests. We think that most people want to volunteer Monday through Friday from 9 to 5, and that is likely true for senior citizens and retirees who make up a large percentage of volunteers in charitable work. Similarly, paid staff would often prefer to work traditional work hours during the week. But what types of volunteers will we engage and attract when we offer volunteer slots in the evenings and weekends? We can recruit people who work during the week and community groups who want to provide community service outside work and school hours.

At Foodshare, we started to expand our volunteer opportunities to additional Saturdays, and they filled up like hotcakes coming off a griddle. Many people are simply not available during traditional work hours: this includes volunteers and also many people who rely on charitable food programs. One of the concerns with providing additional weekend hours was having to pay staff overtime. This is an opportunity to readjust the standard work week, by which some staff work alternative shifts to accommodate programming on the weekend. This is part of reinventing how and when we do our work.

Well-meaning but Potentially Harmful Attitudes

Because many food pantries were created years ago, some of their original founding directors and volunteers have been running the pantry for years. I have noticed that some of these older directors take on the role of matriarch or patriarch over the pantry. This often creates a warm and nurturing environment but can also perpetuate old beliefs and practices because "this is how things have always been done." These types of pantries may be less inclined to offer choice, healthy food, or additional services because they see the mission of the pantry as simply to provide food.

Foodshare recently conducted focus groups with volunteers for our Mobile Foodshare program. We asked for their opinions about how the program operates and some programmatic changes we wanted to make. Despite being designed to allow guests to choose their food, over time many of our distribution locations had volunteers putting food items into clients' bags without choice.

When we discussed the topic of client choice and allowing clients to select their food, one volunteer was very skeptical. He said it wouldn't work. When I asked why, he said it would be challenging for their program because all of the volunteers at this particular site wear t-shirts that say "I Give." I am sure that the t-shirts imply many ways the volunteers are giving back in the community, but they also subtly describe how volunteers were physically giving people food. He said the volunteers were all really proud to wear their shirts and give food to people. It wouldn't work well if clients were choosing their food.

But what is the corresponding t-shirt for people in the food pantry line: "I Get" or "I Receive"? Would you feel proud to wear that t-shirt?

Books such as Sweet Charity?, Toxic Charity, *and* The Stop *all provide examples of volunteers who can perpetuate a model of dependency rather than empowerment.*

I have witnessed examples of volunteers who are well-intentioned and clearly want to help others but who may cause unintentional harm. I have also been influenced by several authors who describe their own experiences with how well-meaning volunteers can cause harm in the charitable food system. Books such as *Sweet Charity?*, *Toxic Charity*, and *The Stop* all provide examples of volunteers who can perpetuate a model of dependency rather than empowerment.

These books are included in the resource list at the end of this chapter, and I highly recommend you read them.

Clients as Volunteers

Often, people who receive food from a food pantry want to volunteer, to provide some sweat equity, and to give back. From my experience, this can work beautifully, but it can sometimes be detrimental, depending on the individual and the circumstances.

When the people who are using a program become a significant portion of the volunteer base, it destroys the division between "us" and "them."

When guests not only receive food from a pantry but also help provide the food as a volunteer, they can help break down divisions between the giver and the receiver. Guests who speak the same language, are from the same community, and experience the same challenges and aspirations as other guests can be great advocates. They can help design the program to be inclusive and address the needs of the community. For example, a guest who serves as a greeter may know people from the community by name and can be a welcoming face. People who receive food from the pantry can tell food pantry directors about cultural food preferences so that the pantry can stock a variety of desirable items that match demand from the community. Food pantries that serve as community food hubs will have spaces where volunteers, guests, and staff can gather to discuss community issues, share resources, and build social capital.

This is a really important point. When the people who are using a program become a significant portion of the volunteer base, it destroys the division between "us" and "them." It will change pantry processes when people getting food are involved in deciding what food should be ordered, how food gets distributed, and when the program should operate. When the people receiving food are also involved with running the program, it will eliminate language and cultural barriers. It will reduce the stigma of coming to get food or other services. The fundamental shifting of power can be done through the volunteer base.

Sarah Kinney, who works at Partnership for a Healthier America and who has spent years working with food pantries, said that in Minnesota it is common practice not to allow food pantry clients to volunteer. Sarah commented that "when we don't involve the community, we won't truly understand or solve the problems we're trying to address. We want to amplify the voices of the people impacted by hunger." Not giving guests the opportunity to volunteer is a missed opportunity to empower food pantry guests and does not create a holistic approach.

However, some guests who serve as volunteers can abuse their power. People who have very little control over their everyday lives can take advantage of their position of "authority" in a food pantry by imposing strict rules. At a recent food pantry distribution, I witnessed a volunteer (who was also a guest) raise her voice at other guests, telling them they had to stop and physically stand on a painted line to wait before they could proceed to get food. She was impatient and rude. This type of behavior can reinforce the shame people feel when going to a food pantry.

Another unintended consequence of guests who serve as volunteers is that they may take extra food or better-quality food before other guests have an opportunity. This causes stress and animosity when guests witness a volunteer who gets preferential treatment.

Training Is Essential

Providing trainings for volunteers at food banks and food pantries is critical because of the valuable roles they play. An initial training and orientation is important, and periodic refresher trainings can be helpful for regular volunteers. It is essential that volunteers understand the mission and values of your organization and how they may have changed over the years. Volunteer trainings and standardized procedures can help to ensure fair treatment for all guests, including those who volunteer, and will reinforce the values you espouse: a welcoming and dignified culture, client choice, diversity and inclusion, healthy food, and a space that is empowering.

The Mount Kisco Interfaith Food Pantry created a volunteer handbook that outlines the pantry's mission, volunteer information, volunteer job duties, and policies and procedures. A link is provided in the resource list at the end of the chapter. The handbook may give you ideas for how to provide orientations for new volunteers or to reorient existing volunteers when you change the way your programs operate. It can be helpful to have some of your seasoned and exceptional volunteers model ideal behavior for new volunteers.

As you read through the examples in this chapter, I encourage you to think about the various volunteers who support your programs and the types of roles and responsibilities they perform. Could they benefit from training to adhere to the values and mission of your organization?

The Role of Volunteers Repurposed

To reinvent the way we provide charitable food (the goal of this book), we will need volunteers. Thankfully, we already have an army. However, you may need to repurpose some of the standard roles for volunteers and the way they spend their time. New initiatives can also create opportunities to engage new volunteers. For example, as we emphasize health and nutrition, volunteers will need to sort through perishable fruits and vegetables that are often messier than cans of food. Determining the nutritional quality of food using a stoplight system like SWAP requires additional volunteer time. Nutrition students and nursing students can help provide nutrition education, rank food nutritionally, and conduct health screenings.

When you shift to a client choice model, volunteers will still spend some time organizing and stocking shelves, but they will no longer pre-bag food. Rather, they will spend more time interacting with guests. Typically, client choice pantries will have volunteers co-shop with clients to help them select food and to help enforce the number of food items a family is allowed to take. Rather than focusing on supervising guests, this can be a great opportunity for volunteers to get to know guests, to ask about each other's family, to share favorite recipes, and to learn what other types of services or programs might be helpful for the guest. When you provide referrals and additional case management services, volunteers will place more emphasis on root causes of hunger and use a strength-based approach when interacting with guests. Social work students can help provide referrals to community services.

As we move to community food hubs that provide holistic services, food pantries will need to establish appointment times and be open several days a week, including some evenings and weekends, and this typically requires additional volunteers. Volunteers will be needed during different days and hours of operation to accommodate working families and to ensure that people do not have to wait in line.

Volunteer Talent—Harnessing Its Potential

Here is an important fact: when volunteer opportunities are centered only on food, they perpetuate the notion that donated food can solve hunger. It won't. Volunteer opportunities that provide experiences of sharing time, listening to others' stories, and understanding the root causes of why someone needs food create bridges. Interactions between volunteers and guests help close the gap between "us" and "them," between economic classes, ages, and races. Breaking down barriers and creating opportunities to connect can also reduce stereotypes, generate new solutions, and build social capital.

Providing volunteer opportunities that are not food related is a way to harness the talent and expertise of volunteers. Let's face it, not everyone wants to sort frozen meat. Think of the other important tasks that must get done to run your food bank or pantry and solicit help with these other vital roles. Some volunteers may be comfortable sorting food but not interacting with clients. That's okay. You can provide a list of available jobs and responsibilities and ask volunteers for their preferences. You can then match interests and skill sets accordingly. Leveraging the talent of volunteers who have skills with social media, graphic design, event planning, accounting, or grant writing will enhance your ability to raise additional funding and perhaps allow you to hire paid staff.

> *Volunteer opportunities that provide experiences of sharing time, listening to others' stories, and understanding the root causes of why someone needs food create bridges.*

Organizational Change

Since you are reading this book, you are likely ready for these types of changes. You're probably already using some of these strategies and are looking for new ideas. But not all of your volunteers or staff members will be thrilled with the new directions. While this chapter focuses on the role of volunteers, this section is also important when thinking about staff throughout your organization. As we discussed in the last chapter, individual behavior change is hard. Organizational change is hard too.

There is a theory called Diffusion of Innovation that helps explain how new ideas spread. The theory describes the phases in which a new idea is shared or communicated to the public and how different groups of people adopt the idea. With a new innovation, some people are early adopters or trendsetters and are willing to try the new idea. The early majority follows quickly after the early adopters. Then there are the middle majority who need more convincing and want to know that the product or program has been well tested before they are willing to try it. Finally, there are others who are slow or resistant to change who are called the laggards.

Malcom Gladwell describes this process brilliantly in his book *The Tipping Point*. He describes various social movements that start slowly with a few early adopters. The change gains momentum with people picking up a new trend, at which point the change reaches a tipping point when the majority of people are using the new program or idea and it becomes mainstream. Finally, the laggards come on board, although some in this later group never choose to adopt the new idea or program.

This can be helpful when you think about your staff and volunteers. Who will serve as your early adopters? You'll want to talk about your new ideas for your food bank or food pantry with the trendsetters who can help champion the change and bring others along. Another way to motivate your staff and volunteers is to visit a local food pantry that is already offering the program you hope to implement, such as a client choice pantry, ask about their experiences, and brainstorm ideas for how you can implement the new idea, program, or system in your organization.

As we reimagine and redesign the way food pantries operate, we will need to communicate these changes and get buy-in from volunteers and staff. When you are considering making a change at your food bank or food pantry, it is important to share the new vision with volunteers and staff to get them onboard. Describe your rationale for making the change, provide evidence and data to show the need, and share the benefit of doing things differently. It is helpful to discuss the new idea early to get feedback from those who will be affected by the change. You can ask volunteers to complete an anonymous survey or hold a team meeting so they can share their ideas, voice their concerns and opinions, and share what they observe working and not working.

Changes—Not Everyone Will Get on Board

When a food bank or food pantry decides to try a new way of operating, embarks on a new program, passes a new policy, or creates a new strategic plan, not everyone is going to like it. As human beings, we generally like to do what is comfortable, what we know, and what we are used to doing. There are many, like the late majority and laggards, who are slow to change. Trying a new path takes strong leadership skills and commitment. And it's worth it.

You may lose some volunteers who do not agree with your new mission, approach, or program and will self-select out. That's okay.

You may lose some volunteers who do not agree with your new mission, approach, or program and will self-select out. That's okay. There may be some volunteers whom you may need to ask not to volunteer at your pantry if they are not aligned with your mission. That's hard but may be necessary for the greater good. Again, think about whether the needs of your volunteers outweigh the needs of your clients.

Take one example from a local food pantry that was using the SWAP stoplight system to promote healthy food. After the pantry had been using SWAP for a number of months, I visited to check in and gather data on their inventory to track changes over time. One of the regular volunteers was noticeably upset about the program. She was literally slamming boxes of food around and audibly sighing in frustration. She said she thought the system was judgmental, that we were acting as the food police and telling clients what they could and could not take from the pantry.

I described my point of view: that I care deeply about client choice and that SWAP is designed specifically for pantries that allow clients to choose their food with dignity. I said SWAP can be a benefit to guests by providing information about which foods are healthier than others: SWAP is a tool to provide information, not to restrict choice. Thankfully, the director of the pantry overheard the conversation, and she came to talk with the volunteer. The director made it clear that the mission of the pantry was not only to provide food for people but to support their health and well-being. She went on to explain that the pantry had made a commitment to using SWAP, and if the volunteer had a problem with this, she should talk with the director. This type of leadership is critical in our charitable food work. We don't want one disgruntled volunteer to sway the opinions and experience of everyone else in a food pantry. It is hard to stand up to a loyal volunteer. I give this director a lot of credit for holding her ground and reiterating the values and mission of the pantry.

It is important to identify the skills and interests of your volunteers to help assign appropriate roles at the food pantry. For example, some volunteers are not comfortable interacting with clients and would prefer behind-the-scene responsibilities. Don't assign them to be a co-shopper in a client choice pantry. If a volunteer wants to be the greeter to hand out numbers and sign people into the pantry, but they don't have great people skills and are often rude to guests, you should reassign them to another role.

If a volunteer has a negative attitude, is not respectful to guests, or is not promoting the mission of a food bank or food pantry, I urge you to find a different role for the volunteer or ask this volunteer to no longer show up for service. I know what you're thinking: "We rely on our volunteers to run our programs, and we could not survive without them. Our volunteers are the lifeblood of our organization. They are volunteering their time, so I can't tell them what to do." I've heard these arguments, but here's the hard truth: we have to remember that the number one priority needs to be serving families struggling with food insecurity, not our volunteers. Stay focused on the mission, culture, and values of your organization and make sure your volunteers model them.

A Response to the Need

Right now I am writing this chapter about volunteers during the unprecedented COVID-19 pandemic. One of the immediate challenges created by COVID-19 was a decline in volunteers. Corporate groups that were scheduled to sort food at food banks cancelled, and senior citizens or others concerned about their health were not able to volunteer. However, the crisis has also brought out compassion and a new flock of volunteers. Many individuals who are out of work, on furlough, or working from home are asking how they can volunteer to ensure that people in their community have enough food.

We conducted brief surveys of our partner programs during COVID-19 to measure the increase in need and to ask how they were adjusting their services. Here is a comment from a food pantry director describing some silver linings of the COVID-19 crisis and how they changed their distribution model. "We have trained a lot of new younger people to do our distribution (our regular crew for client choice are all older retired people). So when we can go back to client choice, we will have several trained back-ups that had not participated before." People are turning crisis into kindness. It's another reflection of how the charitable food system could not exist without the valuable contribution of volunteers and how we can continue to evolve and innovate with changing times.

Action Steps

- Provide trainings on customer service and hospitality for your volunteers to reinforce the mission and values of your organization.
- Conduct a brief anonymous survey with your guests to hear about their experience coming to your program. What do they like and what could be improved about the way they are treated by staff and volunteers?
- Conduct a brief survey with your volunteers to ask what types of expertise they can share beyond food distribution. What do they think is working well and what could be improved with programming? How do they want to be involved in other ways to support guests and your programs?
- If you have a volunteer who has a negative attitude and does not support newer changes, assign them to another program, provide a training to reorient them to your mission, or have a hard conversation about their role in your program. If they are not willing to support your mission, kindly ask them to no longer serve as a volunteer.
- Get creative and think outside the box for new roles for volunteers.
- Hold a volunteer appreciation day to recognize the valuable service provided by your volunteers.
- Set a goal to make one change. I think you're ready.

Resources

Gladwell, Malcom. *The Tipping Point: How Little Things Can Make a Big Difference*. New York: Little, Brown and Company, 2000.

Lupton, Robert. *Toxic Charity: How Churches and Charities Hurt Those They Help (And How to Reverse It)*. New York: HarperOne, 2011.

Mount Kisco Interfaith Food Pantry. "Volunteer Handbook." https://polly -franchini-5sw4.squarespace.com/volunteer-application. [Available as download on volunteer application page.]

Poppendieck, Janet. *Sweet Charity? Emergency Food and the End of Entitlement.* New York: Viking Press, 1998.

Putnam, Robert. "Social Capital Primer." http://robertdputnam.com/bowling -alone/social-capital-primer/.

Saul, Nick, and Andrea Curtis. *The Stop: How the Fight for Good Food Transformed a Community and Inspired a Movement.* Brooklyn, NY: Melville House, 2013.

CHAPTER 9
Evaluation: What Gets Measured Gets Done

One of the things that has always amazed me about the charitable food system is the lack of research conducted to evaluate its impact. Even though there are food banks and food pantries in nearly every community across the country, and these organizations have grown and evolved over five decades, there is very little research to examine how they work. We simply don't evaluate them to determine their effectiveness. With a few exceptions, we turn a blind eye to what happens to the people we serve once they receive their food. We do not measure whether one type of food pantry works better than another. This is unfortunate. I think there are three main reasons why this is so.

First, food pantries were designed to treat an emergency, to fill a short-term gap in resources. We continue to think of food pantries as "emergency" programs that are responding to a short-term situation. We don't evaluate the response to an emergency or natural disaster because we are just trying to get help to people as quickly as possible. For example, if there is a hurricane and people need food, water, and blankets, we bring them food, water, and blankets as quickly as possible. We don't take time to design a study or to collect data. But food pantries are clearly treating a chronic problem and should be evaluated like any other social program. When programs are no longer treating an acute situation, but are now providing services to people for months and often years, yes, it's time to determine which programs are more effective than others.

The second reason I believe we don't evaluate the impact of food pantries is that we as a society really like the idea of giving food to people who are food insecure. Why measure something and turn a critical eye on a program if anecdotally we believe it is a good thing? Many individuals and organizations benefit from the goodwill of "feeding the hungry," so we don't critically look at the effect of our charitable efforts. That's a shame. In his book *Toxic Charity*, Robert Lupton describes the lack of evaluation done in charitable work. He says, "As compassionate people, we have been evaluating our charity by the rewards we receive through service, rather than the benefits received by the served." Even programs that draw on our heartstrings should be evaluated.

Even programs that draw on our heartstrings should be evaluated.

Third, the lack of evaluation in charitable food is also due to how we define success and effectiveness. The main metric used to measure the impact of food banks is pounds of food, which is quick and easy to quantify and report. We may feel like we are evaluating our programs when we simply report the number of pounds distributed. We believe our food pantries are successful and effective if we served a lot of food to a lot of people. For too long we have focused on increasing the numerator (people receiving food) without focusing on reducing the denominator (people who are food insecure). We are busy focused on the short-term goal of providing food. But we also need to step back and look at the big picture of why people need food in the first place and to strategize ways to reduce the number of people who need food.

Typically, we equate effectiveness with efficiency and success with number of pounds distributed. The emphasis on outputs rather than outcomes has limited the scope of research conducted. Thankfully, this is changing, and I'll describe some exciting new research efforts under way.

Measurement of Food Security

In chapter 3, I provided a brief background on how food insecurity was defined and measured starting in the 1980s and early 1990s. Fortunately, we have robust and accurate national information on the number of people who are food insecure and their demographic characteristics. Starting in 1995 and now yearly, the US Census Bureau has collected food security data in collaboration with the USDA. We know that single mothers, Black and Hispanic households, and households with incomes below 100 percent of the poverty line have the highest rates of food insecurity. Female-headed households of color are about twice as likely to experience food insecurity as White female-headed households. This data is extremely valuable because we can track historical trends, compare national prevalence rates with data in our local communities, and target efforts to serve the most vulnerable groups. And we can examine structural and systemic factors that contribute to why these groups in particular are more likely to be food insecure.

For anyone interested in conducting research on food security, you don't have to start from scratch. Use the validated survey tools available through the USDA. I provide links at the end of the chapter. The eighteen-question USDA Food Security Module is the gold standard for measuring food insecurity, and there is also a shorter six-item questionnaire. Both have been validated extensively in various populations.

To further simplify screening, in 2010 the Children's Health Watch developed and validated a two-item questionnaire, called Hunger Vital Sign, based on the USDA module. In 2015 the American Academy of

Pediatrics adopted this screener, recommending that pediatricians use it with all their patients. Clinicians say, "I'm going to read you two statements that people have made about their food situation. For each statement, please tell me whether the statement was often true, sometimes true, or never true for your household in the last twelve months":

1. "We worried whether our food would run out before we got money to buy more."
2. "The food that we bought just didn't last, and we didn't have money to get more."

If a patient says often true or sometimes true to either question, they are considered food insecure.

In addition to the USDA Food Security Module (eighteen-, six-, and two-item questionnaires), Feeding America is encouraging food banks and university partners to use the same validated tools to measure other outcomes. When we use the same measurement tools, we can compare results using apples to apples. For example, the Ending Hunger Community of Practice has identified a couple of useful tools:

- The Lachman Weaver Sense of Control Survey measures self-efficacy—this is the belief in one's ability to make behavior changes, which is a factor for being able to set and reach goals.
- The Consumer Financial Protection Bureau's Financial Wellbeing Scale measures how well a household can pay for and handle expenses—this will help us understand the underlying financial challenges that make it difficult for people to get enough food.

Studies on Food Insecurity

Let me say a few words about types of studies and terminology. The data collected annually for the USDA is cross-sectional data, gathered at one point in time. It provides a snapshot to describe a group of people or a problem. We can use this type of data to report prevalence rates, or the percentage of people who have a certain condition at one time frame. But it doesn't tell us what happens to those people over time. Longitudinal studies, on the other hand, measure the same group of people at different time points to evaluate changes, for example to determine if their food security status or health has improved or if they made fewer economic trade-off decisions.

The largest studies conducted about the charitable food system were the Hunger in America studies, which were cross-sectional studies conducted every four years starting in 1993. The last of these studies, Hunger in America 2014, was the sixth and most comprehensive study in the series, and I've referenced the findings multiple times throughout the book. Results are based on survey data collected from food pantries and meal programs in the Feeding America network and from clients who receive food from those programs. As described on the Hunger in America 2014 website, these studies provide "a profound understanding of the personal and economic circumstances of the households served by the Feeding America network and partner agencies."

Numerous other cross-sectional studies have been conducted in specific communities and particular populations to describe the characteristics of people who are food insecure and who receive food from food pantries. With a few notable exceptions, however, very few longitudinal studies have been conducted to evaluate what happens to people when they receive food from a pantry or whether certain food pantry models are more effective than others in improving health and boosting food security. This is important.

Have you ever wondered what happens to the people who visit food pantries once they go home? How long does the food last? How long until they have to visit the pantry again? Do they feel embarrassed going to the food pantry to get help? Are you looking for ways to measure your work beyond the number of pounds you distribute? Me too.

While we know a lot about who is food insecure and who is most likely to go to food pantries, we know very little about what types of food pantries reduce food insecurity or what impact food pantries have on the health and well-being of those receiving food. We can do better. Without data, it is easy to continue with the status quo and harder to make an argument to change the way we operate.

Fortunately, over the past several years, more academic researchers are entering the field of charitable food security, and several longitudinal studies have been conducted to provide more information about what works. Much of the recent research has focused on the connection between hunger and health. Several studies have evaluated healthy food pantry interventions and measured changes to food security and health outcomes. Feeding America created a website (www.hungerandhealth .feedingamerica.org) to highlight programs, resources, and also research findings about healthy food pantry initiatives. The field of charitable food is ripe for additional research. I welcome faculty members, students, and other researchers to partner with food banks and food pantries, and with me, to evaluate programs. Results will help identify what works and what improvements can be made.

Have you ever wondered what happens to the people who visit food pantries once they go home?

Foodshare Institute for Hunger Research & Solutions

When I joined Foodshare in 2018, I had already been collaborating with various food banks and food pantries around the country and outside the geographic service area of Foodshare. Within one month of my joining Foodshare, my boss, Jason Jakubowski, pitched the bold idea of creating a research institute, a nontraditional department for a food bank, that would provide a platform for conducting research and sharing evidence-based programs. Jason and I dreamed big, and in August of 2019 we took a leap of faith to create the Foodshare Institute for Hunger Research & Solutions. The goal of the Institute is to serve as a resource for other food banks and community partners and to complement and support Feeding America's strategic priorities. The Institute is unique within the Feeding America network and is a prime example of how Foodshare is changing what it means to be a food bank.

Through the Institute, we

1. Develop programs and interventions to decrease food insecurity and promote health and stability;
2. Conduct research to measure the effectiveness of these programs, using both quantitative data collection and qualitative ethical storytelling;
3. Share best practices and evidence-based solutions so others can implement them—we do this via presentations, trainings, webinars, research briefs, and manuals; and
4. Collaborate with multiple partners and funding institutions to advocate for systems change within the charitable food network.

You can check out our website for additional resources and research materials and examples of the tools outlined throughout this book. Please contact us if you are interested in collaborating.

Outputs to Outcomes

The main measure of success for the charitable food system, and what is reported in fundraising appeals, annual reports, and impact statements, is the number of pounds of food distributed each year. Many food banks now describe the number of meals provided, where 1 pound is equal to 1.2 meals, because people can relate more to meals than pounds of food.

For a long time, this type of metric was completely satisfactory for funders and supporters. We could feel satisfied knowing that more people received food. But we can do better. We can measure the nutritional quality of the food provided and measure the impact of what happens to the people who receive the pounds of food.

Many donors are now asking for other examples beyond pounds or meals to show how their money is helping the community.

Many donors are now asking for other examples beyond pounds or meals to show how their money is helping the community. Increasingly, funders are requiring more sophisticated measures to demonstrate outcomes and the impact of programs beyond mere outputs.

So let's be clear about the different terms. Outputs are the products or services we provide, and they describe what we do. Outcomes are the intended benefits, changes, or results we hope to achieve, and they describe why we do our work. Here are a few examples to illustrate the differences:

• Outputs: number of meals distributed, number of SNAP applications submitted, number of backpacks provided to local schools
• Outcomes: increase in "green—choose often" foods distributed, decrease in trade-off decisions between paying for utilities and paying for groceries, increase in food security, reduction in diabetes risk factors, increase in knowledge about local community resources

Because the day-to-day operation of food banks is to collect and distribute food, knowing how many pounds and meals distributed is valuable and will likely always be used as one measure of our work. We can add nuances to show the nutritional quality of the pounds provided and track changes over time.

In 2020, Feeding America adopted new nutrition guidelines developed by Healthy Eating Research for food banks to rank food based on saturated fat, sodium, and sugar. This is really exciting. Rather than just reporting total number of pounds distributed, we can use these guidelines to report the percentage of a food bank's inventory that is "choose often—green," "choose sometimes—yellow," and "choose rarely—red" and measure the changes to these percentages over time. We can also use the data to set benchmarks for increasing the percent of food that is ranked green or yellow and talk with food donors about providing more food that falls into the healthier categories. Currently, the new guidelines are optional and not required by food banks, but Feeding America will be encouraging food banks to start ranking their food. If you're interested in using the new guidelines, you can check out our SWAP stoplight system for tangible tools and resources to rank food and track changes.

A Change in Metrics

While we report on the number of pounds provided, that is not our overall mission or goal. None of us are involved in charitable food work simply to provide food for a couple of days. We want to help people get back on their feet so they do not need to rely on the food pantry. Think about the mission statement of your food bank or food pantry. I would imagine it includes language about ending hunger, changing lives, or engaging your community to build food security. Our metrics should match our end goals. Ultimately, what we measure defines how we view success. And what we measure shapes our values, our programming, how we spend our resources, and our communication strategies. They are interrelated.

Thankfully, many donors are interested in seeing outcomes rather than just outputs. That's good. However, it may be challenging to communicate this paradigm shift to long-time donors who are familiar with the standard measures of success. For example, you likely describe your work as "feeding over 500 people each month," or "providing over 20 million meals last year." You will need language, metrics, and rationale to describe how you are "providing job training, coaching, or nutrition education for 20 people to build their self-sufficiency and diet quality." The former sounds big and tangible. The latter sounds less impressive and takes more time and money.

But here's the thing. Research shows that people who not only receive food at a food pantry but who meet with a coach to work on goals have significant improvements in their food security, ability to make ends meet, their self-efficacy, and their diet quality. Offering More Than Food works. We have scaled and tested the More Than Food program in diverse populations in several different food pantries in three states. It is replicable.

My colleague Marlene Schwartz, the director of the University of Connecticut Rudd Center for Food Policy and Obesity, and I have conducted research on the SWAP stoplight system and found that pantries using SWAP had significant increases in the amount of healthy food available, and customers chose significantly more green food and less red food after SWAP was implemented. A recent study by Christopher Long and colleagues found that food pantries in Arkansas that had nutrition guidelines and that offered client choice had more nutritious food available than nonchoice pantries. These types of evidence-based programs can be highlighted as best practices and replicated by food banks and food pantries. You can include goals in your annual operating plans to measure the number of pantries that provide client choice, provide coaching, and use a nutrition ranking system. We should use evidence and data to inform our work and describe how we are using evidence-based programs to our donors and supporters.

It can be discouraging to think that we are helping only a small number of people with culinary training, coaching, financial savings, or case management. When we are used to telling our supporters and funders

If several food banks or pantries implement the same type of program and use the same measurement tools, we can measure results collectively.

that we provided several million meals' worth of food, it can seem wimpy to describe how we helped fifteen families to become more self-sufficient. Again, it depends on how we measure our success and how we define impact. We should continue to describe the large number of pounds and people served with food for the short-term AND also describe the longer-term outcomes and deeper impact achieved by a smaller number of people who won't need to use the food pantry long-term. When people who receive intensive services become more stable and food secure, they can spread the word so others can receive these holistic services. Over time, the number of people served holistically will grow, and we will have more data to show the longer-term impact of our work.

More food banks and food pantries are providing wraparound services and strategies to promote long-term food security. If we can use standardized approaches and measures, it will help create economies of scale. We can learn from one another and share resources. If several food banks or pantries implement the same type of program and use the same measurement tools, we can measure results collectively. We will also have a larger sample size and statistical power to measure the impact of our programs and to evaluate which ones are effective at building stability and helping people become food secure, as well as which ones sounded good but were not effective and therefore should be revamped or discontinued. If you are interested in conducting research, I would encourage you to network with other food banks to see who is doing similar work and collaborate. I would also encourage you to network with university partners to help evaluate your programs.

What Gets Measured Gets Done

Every year, food banks that are members of the Feeding America network are required to report data to the Feeding America national office as part of the Network Activity Report (NAR). Feeding America then reviews the data and provides a summary report comparing an individual food bank with the entire network of food banks and also to peer food banks with similar demographic features such as size and service area. The reports provide valuable data to show progress year to year and to see how a food bank ranks compared with others. Food banks are required to share the NAR reports with their boards of directors once a year.

One of the key challenges for food banks that want to allocate staff time and resources to progressive holistic work is that the Feeding America network uses pounds of food as its main metric. I applaud Feeding America for its new emphasis on a dual approach of providing food for today while also building food security for the future. But for food banks truly to embrace this approach, the measures of success and what is reported in the NAR need to change.

How we measure our activities and our success matters. As the old saying goes, what gets measured gets done. It will be easier to get organizational buy-in, and to commit staff time for ending hunger strategies, if food banks are required to report these types of activities yearly and see how they compare with other food banks. There's nothing like a little friendly competition to challenge organizations to set and meet new goals.

A Measure for Capacity Building

Throughout this book, I have described several best practices for food pantries, including providing a dignified culture with short wait times and client choice, promoting healthy food, and offering wraparound services. These are programmatic initiatives, but we can also apply a research lens to gather data to understand to what degree food pantries are offering these programs and then measure changes over time to build capacity.

At Foodshare, we created a survey as part of our annual renewal application for partner programs. In addition to standard questions about their infrastructure, we included questions about offering a welcoming culture, healthy client choice, and connection to community resources. We view these practices along a continuum. We applied the Stages of Change theory and asked about how ready they were to focus on these topics, what they perceived as barriers to implementing them, and then asked detailed questions about their current programming in each area.

One thing I have found is that if you ask food pantries if they offer client choice, the vast majority will say yes. But we have to be careful of thinking of this as a simple yes/no question, because there are varying degrees of choice. And they matter. We ask how food is distributed at the food pantry and measure choice on a scale from 1 to 5 as follows:

1. Food is packed in bags or boxes before clients arrive. Each client is given a bag or box to take home. (No choice)
2. Clients receive a prepacked bag of food, and then they can choose a few items from a "choice" selection. (Limited choice)
3. Clients tell volunteers what food items they want, sometimes from a menu, and volunteers then pack in a bag or box for the client. (Modified choice)
4. Clients can see food options and can select what they want. Clients pack their food in a bag or box. (Full choice)
5. Clients can see food options, select what they want, and pack their own bag or box. Additionally, pantry volunteers assist clients in selecting healthy food options. (Full healthy choice)

As you can see, there are subtle but important differences between each level of choice. We rank pantries on a scale from 1 (low capacity) to 5 (high capacity) based on this question and several others to determine the degree to which they were incorporating the best practices of healthy client choice, connection, and culture at the food pantry.

We are now using the data to inform our work. When our partner program staff talk with pantry directors or go on site visits, they can use the information to make suggestions to help the pantry move along the continuum to the next level of programming. Information about a pantry's readiness for change and current programming helps to meet the pantries where they are and target services rather than applying a one-size-fits-all approach. For example, if a director described lack of refrigeration as a barrier to promoting healthier food, they would be

Information about a pantry's readiness for change and current programming helps to meet the pantries where they are and target services rather than applying a one-size-fits-all approach.

encouraged to apply for a small grant from the food bank for equipment. If the pantry is interested in offering client choice, but they say space is a barrier, our staff can brainstorm ways to reconfigure the layout or the pantry hours to accommodate more choice.

We will conduct the survey again within two years to measure changes along the scale to see what improvements have been made and where we need to target additional support. For example, if a food pantry scored a 2 for client choice, next year we would want to see them score at least a 3 by offering more opportunities for guests to choose their food. I am also collaborating with the Worcester County Food Bank in Massachusetts to use the assessment and build the capacity of a sample of their food pantry network. We conducted the survey and asked if pantries were interested in receiving trainings and support to offer more client choice, to provide referrals and coaching, or to provide a more welcoming culture. We can use the data to help pantries move along the scale and monitor their changes.

Many food banks within the Feeding America network gather data to tier or segment their food pantries and meal programs. Often the tiers are based on number of pounds and people served but can also include whether the pantry has paid staff, whether it provides other services, and how engaged the pantry is with the food bank. This process of gathering data can be valuable to

- Highlight superstar pantries that can serve as role models for others,
- Identify underperforming pantries,
- Provide trainings and resources to build capacity of lower-tier pantries,
- Create minimum guidelines for new pantries to join the network, and
- Allocate resources to align with the food bank's overall mission.

For example, the Maryland Food Bank conducted a network restructuring project. They performed an analysis to understand gaps in service that limited their ability to address hunger throughout Maryland. They used the data to create four groups of agencies within their network. The goal was to build the capacity of agencies within their network, and prioritize where the food bank allocated staff time to support the higher-tier agencies.

Data Collection and Research

Many people get intimidated by the idea of research. They think it has to be complicated, expensive, and time consuming. But it doesn't have to be. There are many ways to get started gathering data that don't have to be overwhelming. Think about it this way: gathering information about the people who participate in our programs, and about the types of programs that we run, can help us understand our work better and know where we can make improvements. Knowledge is power. New technology and programs make it easier and cheaper to collect and analyze data. We can use the information, data, and evidence to help inform our work and make our programs better. Having data can also help with fundraising to garner new or bigger funding sources. How about that for added incentive?

Typically, when we think about research we think about quantitative studies, using numerical data, charts, and tables. Quantitative research is really valuable, but a great way to embark on research and start gathering input from your community is through qualitative research. This can involve asking open-ended questions through structured interviews with individual stakeholders or in a group setting via focus groups. By use of open-ended questions (rather than yes/ no or multiple choice questions), qualitative data helps gather information about opinions, motivations, and perceptions about a topic. You should ask the same questions in the interviews and focus groups to keep them standardized and to identify themes. You want to conduct interviews and focus groups until you reach "saturation," the point at which you are hearing the same information from various respondents and not gaining new insights.

> *Qualitative research is a great way to understand how people talk about a topic, what they perceive as the strengths and limitations with current programming, and what they suggest for improvements.*

Qualitative research is a great way to understand how people talk about a topic, what they perceive as the strengths and limitations with current programming, and what they suggest for improvements. You can identify common themes and highlight relevant quotes to describe the problem you hope to address and the programs you hope to implement. You can also use this information to develop quantitative survey questions.

For example, when we were developing the SWAP stoplight system, we started with focus groups. We had identified six food pantries that were willing to pilot the new nutrition program, and we wanted their opinions on the language used for the stoplight and also about challenges they envisioned with implementing the system. They liked the health focus, to be able to label foods as diabetes friendly, and they liked the language of choose often, sometimes, and rarely. They also told us it would be very hard to start the program during the holidays of Thanksgiving and Christmas and that we would need to train their volunteers so it could be sustainable. We used their feedback to develop signage, to determine the timing of launching the program, and to provide training materials for staff and volunteers.

Research Goals and Relevant Questions

As you consider evaluating a project, start by thinking through your overall study goals. What do you want to know about your program or the people you are serving? Get clear on your main research goal. Make sure that the research goals are practical and within the scope of your organization so that you will be able to act upon the results. Make sure the questions you ask in interviews or surveys will help you answer your main research objective. Because time is limited, you want to keep your interview or survey short, so you want to ask the right questions.

Think about who you need to study to help answer your research question. This could include community partners, food pantry staff, or food pantry guests. Make sure the people you include in your study represent the people who participate in a given program, not just one segment. Consider how much time you will need to prepare materials and gather the data and what staff, volunteers, or student interns will need to be involved. After you have your data, you'll need to analyze it and report what you learned. A university or research partner can be helpful with many of these steps.

As we reinvent the way we provide charitable food, we will start to use new metrics and measures of our success, from pounds to people. As we help connect people to services and supports, we can measure the decrease in number of people coming to the food pantry on a chronic basis or the number of people who enrolled in SNAP, health insurance, job training, nutrition education, and so on. This will require the ability to gather information about the people we serve and to track their experiences over time. Many food banks are using software programs such as Oasis or Link2Feed to track this type of data.

The research team at Feeding America has developed a client survey with a standard set of questions to help food banks gather data about the people they serve and with separate modules that focus on various topics. That way a food bank can select a shorter version of the survey to measure basic information and add modules to study additional topics, such as housing stability, disability, diet quality, and coping strategies. These efforts are major advances for the field of charitable food work and will help us to understand the people we are serving (to help reduce stereotypes and create empathy) and to evaluate the impact of our services (to measure changes over time to see what works and what was not very effective).

As we reinvent the way we provide charitable food, we will start to use new metrics and measures of our success, from pounds to people.

Community–University Partnerships

There are many opportunities for collaboration between food bank and food pantry staff and local universities and research centers. If you want to gather data and conduct research but don't know how to start, or if you are starting a new program and want to evaluate it, contact a local university to see if they would be willing to collaborate with you. Often, academic researchers, particularly graduate students, are looking for research topics and community sites for conducting research.

A word of caution about what we want to avoid. Food banks or food pantries without much research experience can run the risk of conducting research without sound methodology and can report results that are potentially misleading. On the other extreme, academic institutions can conduct "helicopter research" whereby academic teams do not consult with community groups before or after the research is done. University staff swoop into a community, collect data, return to the university to analyze the data, and write academic journal articles and community groups never see the results of the work and are not included in the process.

Ideally, universities and food banks can partner on research projects that will be mutually beneficial. Food bank or food pantry staff can approach the university with a specific research project or research question. Or academic members can reach out to a food bank or pantry and ask with what types of research projects they would like help. This allows the researchers to have access to a community site for data collection, and they can use the data for thesis projects and published journal articles. Food banks and pantries can receive valuable data that they may not otherwise be able to collect or analyze.

At the beginning of any community–university partnership, all partners should agree on some basic ground rules. Often, nonprofits and academics use different terminology and may seem to speak different languages, so you want to make sure you understand the parameters of the research project. Discuss the scope of the project and the types of research questions you want answered. Talk about the time frame and resources that will be involved. From the food bank's perspective, you don't want to wait two years before you see results. The research partner should be able to provide preliminary data and short research briefs describing the results to show progress. I am a fan of creating research briefs with quantitative data (numbers and statistics) and qualitative data (quotes and stories) that can tell a compelling story. This helps translate the research results into practice. Food banks and pantries can use the research briefs to inform their programming, to provide reports to their board of directors, or to include with grant proposals.

Program Evaluation

The idea of evaluation may seem judgmental, and some people may fear doing research if it may show flaws in a program we love. But the point is to make a good program even better. This was the case with the Mobile Food-share program, which is a pantry-on-wheels that brings fresh produce and other food to those in need at over sixty community sites throughout Greater Hartford, Connecticut. Like many other food banks, we started our mobile program because we had access to fresh produce, but our partner programs were not equipped to handle perishables because they lacked refrigerators or equipment. Our Mobile Foodshare program has grown over eighteen years and is our largest and most visible program in the community. Historically, the program operates Monday through Friday from 9 a.m. to 3 p.m.

In 2018, we conducted a comprehensive program review to better understand the program's strengths and opportunities for improvement and to assure that this flagship program was aligned with Foodshare's current organizational mission, vision, and values.

In 2018, we conducted a comprehensive program review to better understand the program's strengths and opportunities for improvement and to assure that this flagship program was aligned with Foodshare's current organizational mission, vision, and values. The review involved staff interviews, focus groups with site coordinators, a survey of Mobile Foodshare clients, and a good look at our internal structure and operations.

We found that the program is effective at bringing millions of pounds of healthy food to people in need through local community partnerships. But we also found there were some inefficient delivery routes, poorly managed sites, and some duplication in sites. We restructured the schedule and eliminated a few sites. We identified a need for new trainings with site coordinators to reinforce expectations and best practices. The trainings discuss the role of volunteers, creating a welcoming environment, conflict resolution, handling complaints, and client choice.

To gather client feedback, we chose a representative sample of twenty-five sites (e.g., urban and rural, with different drivers, small and large attendance). We conducted a survey of our Mobile Foodshare guests over the course of about four weeks. We invited people to participate in the survey while they were waiting in line for food before and during distributions. The survey was available in English and Spanish and also in Polish in certain sites. In total, 1,956 people participated.

We did this old-school by creating a one-page survey and administered the survey with paper and pen. We found that only 28 percent of the participants had a child under age eighteen in the household, while more than half of participants (64 percent) reported having at least one person over age sixty in the household. Less than one in five respondents (19 percent) said someone in their household was employed. What we found was that the Mobile Foodshare program was doing a good job serving families with seniors and people who are unemployed but relatively few working families or those with kids. In addition, over half of respondents said they know people who need food but could not attend the mobile site.

We then piloted our Mobile Foodshare program on Saturdays to provide food on the weekends. On average, 76 percent of Saturday Mobile Foodshare attendees reported that they were new to Mobile Foodshare. The traditional program is convenient for routine operations of the food bank, including staff time and schedules, but was not reaching vulnerable people in the community. Through our review, we recommended areas for improvement, such as having a Spanish-speaking driver for certain sites to better serve Hispanic customers. This is an example of the need to continuously review how services are provided, to examine who we are serving and who we may be missing, and then to correct course.

Many nonprofit organizations, and particularly volunteer-run organizations, simply don't have the resources to conduct a formal study. I would encourage you to partner with a research organization, a local university, or with Foodshare's Institute for Hunger Research & Solutions to help evaluate your work. Sometimes even well-funded organizations do not want to take the time or additional resources to evaluate their work. It can be easier to continue with the status quo. When many people need food, it can be tempting to just keep running the same program year after year. But by conducting even some basic reviews, we gain valuable insights into the strengths and weaknesses of our programs and what could be improved. Gathering data can help food banks to reinforce best practices and to build the capacity of our network to better serve the people in our communities. We can take the good work we are doing and make it even better.

Action Steps

- Review your mission statement and the metrics you use to describe success. Think about the outputs and outcomes you measure and report and make sure they align with your mission.
- Start with qualitative research by conducting interviews or focus groups.
- Create a community–university partnership to evaluate charitable food programs.
- At the food pantry level, ask the people you serve for their feedback about the food and services you provide. You can conduct focus groups or gather brief surveys.
- At the food bank level, measure the capacity of your partner programs and measure changes over time. Use the data to target additional trainings and resources to build capacity.
- At the Feeding America level, include additional metrics in the Network Activity Report that reflect the progressive focus of addressing root causes of hunger.
- Take one step toward change.

Resources

Children's Health Watch. "Hunger Vital Sign." https://childrenshealthwatch.org/public-policy/hunger-vital-sign/.

Cooksey-Stowers, Kristen, Katie Martin, and Marlene B. Schwartz. "Client Preferences for Nutrition Interventions in Food Pantries." *Journal of Hunger & Environmental Nutrition* 14, no. 1–2 (2018): 18–34. https://doi.org/10.1080/19320248.2018.1512929.

Cooksey-Stowers, Kristen, Margaret Read, Michele Wolff, Katie Martin, Michelle McCabe, and Marlene B. Schwartz. "Food Pantry Staff Attitudes about Using a Nutrition Rating System to Guide Client Choice." *Journal of Hunger &*

Environmental Nutrition 14, no. 1–2 (2018): 35–49. https://doi.org/10.1080/19320248.2018.1512930.

Feeding America. *Hunger in America 2014.* https://www.feedingamerica.org/research/hunger-in-america.

Feeding America. "Map the Meal Gap." https://map.feedingamerica.org/.

Hunger + Health/ Feeding America. https://hungerandhealth.feedingamerica.org.

More Than Food. "Foodshare Institute for Hunger Research & Solutions." http://site.foodshare.org/site/PageServer?pagename=institute.

US Department of Agriculture Economic Research Service. "Food Security Measurement Tools." Food Security in the U.S. https://www.ers.usda.gov/topics/food-nutrition-assistance/food-security-in-the-us/measurement.aspx.

CHAPTER 10
Structural Inequalities and Systems Change

In the preface of the book, I promised a roadmap for designing food pantries that are relational and emphasize social justice and equity. A big part of this journey toward transformational food pantries is addressing injustices across racial, gender, and class lines. These are complex issues and challenging things to discuss, particularly for White Americans and men. It requires tough conversations between marginalized and privileged groups.

Let me introduce the elephant that just walked into the room. When we decide to take a stand against racial inequality and to advocate for progressive policies that reduce systemic injustices, we need to be prepared that we may turn off some of our long-time supporters and donors. And perhaps some staff and volunteers. The roadmap to ending hunger is paved with justice, but it is not an easy ride.

I am by no means an expert on racial equity or diversity. But I know how critically important it is to talk about these subjects if we are to move our charitable food network forward. I want to be in the arena, not on the sidelines. I approach these subjects with humility and with an open mind, ears, and heart—and with the courage to address controversial topics, and probably screw up, and get back up again and keep trying. I hope you'll join me in the arena.

Systemic Inequality

Have you ever pulled yourself up by your bootstraps? Do you even know what that means? I've never really been able to picture the metaphor. But I do know that it is harder for some groups to pull themselves up than others, particularly if they don't have any bootstraps, so to speak. My colleague Dr. Kristen Cooksey-Stowers, who is an assistant professor of Health Disparities at the University of Connecticut, says, "Some groups pull themselves up by their bootstraps and are then kicked back down."

But let's be clear, food insecurity is not caused by a lack of food but a lack of political will by policy makers and decision makers. It is caused by systemic injustices, structural racism, and unequal privilege.

When we think about hunger, we typically think of an individual's behavior or a family's tough plight. Yet data consistently show that there are certain groups of people who are at higher risk of food insecurity than others. Single mothers with children have the highest rates of food insecurity, along with Black and Hispanic households. There are historical, social, and political reasons why these particular groups are more likely to live in poverty and become food insecure. In order to build long-term food security and help individuals achieve the American dream, we need to remove structural barriers.

Hunger in America has long been viewed as a nonpartisan issue. When we define the problem as simply a lack of food, it is easy to rally support from politicians, corporations, and individuals to provide food for "the hungry." But let's be clear, food insecurity is not caused by a lack of food but a lack of political will by policy makers and decision makers. It is caused by systemic injustices, structural racism, and unequal privilege.

When we realize that being food insecure is not just about an individual's choices, we are more likely to advocate for broader policy and system changes. In this chapter, we will explore ways to focus on root causes of hunger both by working closely with individuals who have been historically marginalized or historically oppressed and by advocating for broader policy changes. Because we need both approaches. This will help us move from charity to justice. Charity highlights differences between the giver and the receiver, whereas justice helps create equity and unity among different groups of people.

A Long History of Discrimination

The four hundredth anniversary of slavery in the United States was marked in 2019. Understanding our history and the ramifications of centuries of social policies is important for understanding our current state of unequal access to food, income inequality, and health disparities between Whites and Blacks and other people of color.

In 2020, the murders of George Floyd, Breonna Taylor, and Ahmaud Arbery, three unarmed Black individuals, highlighted how pervasive racism continues to be in our society. These tragic events sparked an outcry for racial justice and calls to action for drastic reforms, not only for police accountability but also structural changes in housing, prison reforms, and changes to the criminal justice system, to name just a few. I think part of the reason these deaths struck such a collective nerve was because news stories were already highlighting how people of color were more likely to be infected, diagnosed, and die from COVID-19 and more likely to lose their jobs because of COVID-19 before we watched the video of George Floyd's murder. These events have spurred an incredible new awareness about White privilege and structural racism.

Our country has a long history of discrimination against Blacks, and more recently Hispanic and immigrant families, regarding employment, banking, and home ownership. Just one poignant example is how millions of Black WWII veterans were denied access to loans through the GI bill. These people fought bravely for our country, but owing to bias and discriminatory practices, they were not eligible to receive loans and apply for mortgages in newly formed suburban towns. The ripple effects of this are long lasting and helped contribute to racially segregated communities and the widening gap in wealth, education, and opportunity.

Discrimination against women regarding education and employment opportunities manifests in continued undervaluing of traditionally female jobs and the persistent gender pay gap, or the difference between the earnings of men and women. Women now receive more graduate degrees than men and have made strides in moving up the corporate ladder and into male-dominated job fields. Yet according to PayScale, women made only $0.81 for every dollar a man made in 2020. Women of color earn 25 percent less than White men, or $0.75 for every dollar.

Structural racism and gender bias make it harder for female-headed households and people of color to get decent paying jobs, to attend high-quality schools, to save money, and to buy homes. Institutional policies that discriminate against women and people of color create an uneven playing field. These historical events have played a tremendous role in creating what we call the root causes of hunger and the social determinants of health. The gap in wealth and opportunity expands over time and over generations. According to the Federal Reserve, Black Americans own about one-tenth of the wealth of White Americans. The net worth (assets minus debt) of a typical White family was $171,000 compared with $17,000 for a typical Black family in 2016.

When we see that single moms and Black and Hispanic households are most likely to be food insecure, it is a reflection of these historic injustices.

When we see that single moms and Black and Hispanic households are most likely to be food insecure, it is a reflection of these historic injustices. When we understand the underlying disparities in income and opportunity, it can help build empathy and help us avoid blaming people of color if they lack individual success. Rather, we can look to organizational, systemic, and policy solutions in order to help all people reach their full potential.

The Role of White Privilege

In the United States, we love the image of the American dream in which individual effort leads to success. However, if you are White, you might not recognize the privilege you hold simply by the color of your skin. You may not appreciate the quality of your schools and may take for granted your ability to get a bank account to safely save your money or a loan to buy a house. When we fail to recognize the structural factors that have paved the way for our lot in life, we run the risk of thinking our achievements are solely due to our individual merits—and, conversely, thinking that people who have not achieved as much are not as intelligent or as hardworking. This can lead to implicit bias of seeing people of color as less worthy or deserving.

Talking about White privilege makes many White people uncomfortable. But like many issues we're discussing in this book, in order to have transformational change, we need to get out of our comfort zones, to be vulnerable, and confront challenging topics. It is not enough to say that people of color are at a disadvantage. We need to recognize the corollary fact that being White has advantages. We need to examine closely the privileges that Whites possess simply by waking up White and dismantle barriers for people of color. This will help us make progress toward not only understanding why people of color are disproportionately food insecure but finding ways to create more equity.

These topics may seem far afield from our conversations about food access. But police brutality is just one example of a systemic injustice that makes it harder for people of color to afford basic necessities. Unequal treatment of certain groups of people, whether in lending policies, hiring practices, or racial profiling create income inequality, which leads to food insecurity. Having a firm understanding of structural racism is key to food banks and food pantries providing charitable food in ways that are relational and trauma informed and that emphasize social justice as part of their mission. Since we didn't learn about these issues in our high school history classes, now is a great time to read up and learn more. Many great resources and books have been highlighted in the wake of the George Floyd murder to raise awareness, and I've included a couple at the end of the chapter.

Low-Income Workers and Food Insecurity

Think about the people who clean the dishes at your favorite restaurant, those who take care of your kids at daycare, who work in hotels and nursing homes, and even who work in the warehouse of your local food bank. The United Way developed a project to help understand the struggles of people like this who work full-time but cannot afford basic necessities. The United Way calls the population ALICE, which stands for Asset-Limited, Income-Constrained, Employed. In other words, the working poor. ALICE describes an individual who is not living below the poverty line but who is likely to be food insecure. They may not qualify for federal food assistance programs like SNAP because their income is too high, but their income is too low to cover necessary expenses, including food.

The United Way calls the population ALICE, which stands for Asset-Limited, Income-Constrained, Employed. In other words, the working poor.

Millions of Americans are working but do not receive benefits, do not have paid medical leave, and do not have enough food for their family. This doesn't align with the bootstrap theory and American dream. The United Way's ALICE project helps spur community conversations and build new partnerships between schools, corporations, employers, and government agencies to advocate for policy changes to support low-wage families. At Foodshare, we introduced the ALICE project to our whole staff during a monthly meeting, and several people commented that it gave them a better appreciation for the people we serve.

Even before the COVID-19 health crisis, the Federal Reserve documented that 40 percent of Americans did not have adequate savings to withstand an unexpected $400 expense. Millions of Americans are living on a razor-thin margin with very little safety net. Many people who were severely impacted by COVID-19 are part of the ALICE population. Just one or two paychecks away from needing help. People who lost their jobs during the pandemic are much more likely to be people of color and those with no college education. Kristen Cooksey-Stowers describes how hurricane Katrina exposed the "cumulative barriers posed by Blackness and income disparities" between neighborhoods in New Orleans. Similarly, COVID-19 revealed deep inequalities for people who are vulnerable not just to job loss but also to the virus itself.

Nancy Roman, the CEO of Partnership for a Healthier America, stated that "COVID-19 has caused historic disruption and also brought insight and clarity. One glaring truth it has exposed is gross inequity throughout the food system at every level. Poor diets that have caused and exacerbated obesity, diabetes, heart disease, and other diet-related chronic diseases are partly responsible for higher death rates among communities of color and those facing poverty." The combination of the pandemic and the most recent killings of Black Americans by police have raised awareness about income inequality and systemic injustices that create disparities in both health and wealth.

Bridges Out of Poverty

Several years ago, I had the opportunity to attend a poverty conference in Ohio, a three-day event where experts spoke about trends and metrics for measuring poverty and examples of policies that were helping to alleviate poverty. It was enlightening to attend a conference filled with people who all cared about the issue of poverty and were working hard to find ways to reduce it. Researchers presented sophisticated charts of income trends over the past few decades. Analysts provided recommendations for policy changes that would effectively address poverty.

But my favorite part of the conference was a presentation about Bridges Out of Poverty and the companion program called "Getting Ahead in a Just-Gettin' By World." Bridges was developed by Ruby Payne, and Getting Ahead is a workshop and curriculum that was developed by Ruby Payne, Phil DeVol, and Terie Dreussi Smith. The Bridges framework provided a lot of aha moments for me (and their publishing company is aptly named the aha! Process). Many of the lessons and fundamental tenets of Bridges have informed my work with food pantries, especially in our More Than Food program.

Just as it is hard to talk about racism and White privilege, talking about social class also makes us uncomfortable. We like the idea that most Americans are comfortably part of the middle class. It seems impolite and awkward to talk about socioeconomic status, the combination of income, education, and employment that determine whether you live in upper, middle, or lower class.

But if we want to help build opportunities for people to be food secure and get out of poverty, it is helpful to understand the different perspectives of people from the different socioeconomic classes of poverty, middle class, and wealth. Bridges Out of Poverty describes how people in each economic class have skills, but some of these skills are more highly valued than others. People in poverty are much more resilient than we give them credit for. It takes a lot of work to make ends meet with limited resources. However, schools, businesses, and institutions, which are necessary for getting out of poverty, operate from middle class norms.

Bridges Out of Poverty includes various constructs to describe differences between classes. For example, when you're living in poverty, the focus is on survival, and relationships are critical to help you survive. The driving forces for those in middle class are work, education, and achievement. When you meet someone new, a typical middle class question is, "What do you do?" For those living in wealth, the driving forces are financial, political, and social connections. It's like the old adage "It's not necessarily what you know, but who you know."

Not being able to plan for one's future is what poverty feels like.

COVID-19 gave us all an understanding of what it's like to live with uncertainty, including not knowing when you'll be able to get toilet paper. Not being able to plan for one's future is what poverty feels like. If you are living in poverty, the environment is often chaotic and unstable, so people have to focus on solving immediate, concrete problems. The time horizon for people in poverty is about two days, for middle class it is two years, and for those in wealth it is about two decades.

We can use this understanding of different views of time when we design our charitable food programs. When food pantries are open for two hours twice a month, it can be challenging and stressful for people living in poverty. Having flexible days of the week for appointments will be less stressful for food pantry guests. Setting up appointments can provide a dignified shopping experience so people don't need to wait in line, but you can also build in extra flexibility to accommodate hectic schedules.

Middle class values focus on efficiency, but this can hinder the ability to focus on relationships, a key value for those in poverty. Trying to hand out food as quickly as possible may seem like a very efficient system from a middle class point of view, but setting up the food distribution with a longer schedule can create a more relaxed atmosphere and time to say a few words as customers shop. Getting right to the agenda at the beginning of a meeting may seem efficient, but building relationships means taking a few minutes for small talk and hearing about someone's family. Think about ways to structure your services to allow time and space for building relationships.

The Program "Getting Ahead"

Getting Ahead is a sixteen-session program designed for individuals who are struggling with poverty to investigate some of the harsh realities of where their life is today, where they want to be, and how they can set goals to build self-sufficiency to get ahead. I love the intentional word choices for the Getting Ahead program. Facilitators lead the structured workshop and eight to ten "investigators" use workbooks to map out their social network, to create a budget, and to set goals for getting ahead. The participants are called investigators because they are exploring the impact that poverty has had on them in order to create a plan for becoming self-sufficient—their "future story." The facilitators do not tell participants what to do or instruct them; they simply enable the discussion.

The Getting Ahead curriculum and accompanying workbook describe some of the systemic injustices, like payday lenders, that can make it hard for individuals to save money. The program helps empower individuals to become advocates for their own well-being but also to address injustices in their community. Investigators have raised their voices to advocate for larger policy changes, like an increase in the minimum wage and more convenient bus routes.

Several years ago, Foodshare piloted the Getting Ahead program, and I helped to train facilitators. One of our investigators commented, "This program has helped me to begin to understand what poverty is and how it affects me, my family, and my community. It has helped me to take total charge of my life without being swayed by outside negative opinions. Learning to set boundaries for my life and prioritize everyday activities so that I can get ahead not only for myself but for the people around me."

The Value of Social Capital

For individuals who live in families and communities that have struggled with structural inequalities and generational poverty, where few people have finished college and the majority have relied on government assistance, it can be hard to buck the norm. One of the big aha moments from the Bridges work for me was realizing that in order to get ahead, individuals will have to let go of at least one important relationship, at least temporarily. Close family members and friends may not understand the goals and dreams of someone trying to advance out of poverty. This is hard because, as I mentioned, relationships are a core value and necessary asset to survive in poverty.

Think of these scenarios. Whenever Joe hangs out with his neighbor, he tends to do something stupid and finds himself in trouble. Joe likes hanging out with his neighbor, but in order to keep his job, Joe makes the conscious decision to not spend Friday nights with him. Sherry wants to enroll in community college so she can get a better job. It will be difficult to work full-time and take night classes, but she is committed to making a better life for herself and her kids. However, Sherry's mom questions why she thinks she's better than the rest of the family. She says Sherry is trying to live beyond her means. In order to improve her education, Sherry decides to find a friend to watch her kids when she's in school instead of relying on her mom.

In his book *Hillbilly Elegy*, J. D. Vance describes the difficulty of moving from one social class to another. Growing up poor in Appalachian Ohio, his family valued loyalty, but he witnessed many people getting stuck in a cycle of poverty and dependency. He had to buck against cultural beliefs and norms to succeed in school. He describes the complicated process of moving from poor, working class, White Appalachia to the middle class and attending Yale Law School.

> *In order to help people move out of poverty, we need to create opportunities for individuals from different racial and economic classes to meet and interact.*

In order to help people move out of poverty, we need to create opportunities for individuals from different racial and economic classes to meet and interact. Designing food pantries as community food hubs where people come for food but also connection and socializing will help bridge social capital. Create space and opportunities for food pantry guests to interact with volunteers, staff, and other food pantry guests. Appreciating the different mindsets and skill sets of people in low, middle, and upper classes can give us empathy and appreciation for how to help people transition out of poverty. This will help everyone gain exposure to different cultural values associated with class. Knowing people outside your immediate social circle and economic class can be the difference between getting ahead and just getting by. Who you know matters.

Soft Skills

In their compelling article "Poverty and the Controversial Work of Nonprofits," Jindra and Jindra argue that while we need to change policies and the broader system (structural racism, lack of livable wages), in the meantime we also need to focus on relational work to help individuals help themselves. This involves changing habits, reducing stress, and building social capital. They argue, "Mere job training often won't do it, since soft skills are also crucial. As part of the process, this requires digging into sensitive areas of class and culture, and of giving people the tools that most of the middle class already has."

What do we mean by soft skills? Examples include what to wear to an interview, how to answer the phone professionally, how to create a resume, sending a thank you note after a job interview, making sure to contact your employer if you are running late for work, setting up an email account, and setting up a banking account. If you grow up in the middle class, your parents and neighbors have modeled these behaviors for you. They seem normal and part of your culture. If you grow up in poverty, you may not have these skills, but they are essential stepping stones for building food security. We can help the people we serve by acknowledging not only the skills and positive values of surviving in poverty but also the role modeling skills and coping strategies required in middle class institutions.

If we overlook these soft skills and inherent differences between growing up in middle class versus in poverty, we can remain stuck in providing basic needs of food rather than transformational tools to build self-sufficiency. I would encourage you to use the ALICE framework and Bridges Out of Poverty concepts, and materials on structural racism and White privilege, to have conversations with various stakeholders in your organization and your community about economic class. This should involve businesses, colleges, banks, and other nonprofits to discuss the systemic injustices and inequalities that keep people in poverty. This is not always comfortable. You may need to channel your inner badass to have these difficult conversations. Creating a shared language about economic class will help us design programs that help individuals move from one class to another.

Upstream Approaches for Systems Change

You've probably heard of the classic fish analogy: if you give a man a fish, he will eat for a day. This is the model of traditional food pantries that provide a short-term supply of food and little else. In these settings, it is very likely that people will need to rely on the pantry on a chronic basis. People are grateful for the food, but it can also lead to dependency because it is designed as a short-term solution.

The analogy continues that if you teach a man to fish, he will eat for a lifetime. The idea is that if we can provide information and teach skills, then people will have the necessary resources to become food secure and will not need to rely on the food pantry long-term. We like this analogy because it represents the American philosophy that providing education is what is required to help people make better choices. It also reflects our belief that if people just pull themselves up by their bootstraps and start fishing, they will have enough food. The Getting Ahead workshops and our More Than Food program focus on providing resources and motivation to help people set goals and build skills for stability, health, and longer-term food security.

But the fish analogy shouldn't stop there, and neither should our work. Because it implies that everyone has access to fishing poles, that the water is clean, and that there is an ample supply of fish. To translate, we think that if we just teach someone how to get a job, then they will successfully apply for a job, start working, and be able to provide for their family. But we know it is more complicated than that. Systems change is often required, and a safety net of additional supports is needed to build true self-sufficiency: things like living wages, affordable child care and health care, and access to transportation. Even when individuals are doing their best to work and take care of their family, we need to ensure an adequate safety net is in place to support them. This requires a systems approach, not just information.

In *Toxic Charity*, Robert Lupton writes, "What good is job training if the available jobs won't enable a man to support his family? If we are to teach people to both fish and thrive, we must figure out how to make use of the lake's potential." For example, nutrition education is helpful to explain the benefits of eating vegetables, whole grains, and lean proteins. But systems change is often required to ensure that our food banks and food pantries provide these items and that local grocery stores have these items available at reasonable prices. Similarly, a budgeting class or financial literacy workshop can provide valuable tools to help people manage their money. But it can be hard to budget and save if you don't have enough money for the minimum balance required to set up a bank account.

Access to Banks

Building on the fish analogy above, even if people are trying to fish, the water can be filled with sharks. Compared with higher-income neighborhoods, low-income communities and communities of color have more predatory services such as check-cashing businesses, payday lenders, and rent-to-own shops that charge exorbitant interest rates. These businesses prey upon low-income families and keep people from getting ahead.

According to a 2017 survey by the Federal Deposit Insurance Corporation, 25 percent of US households were unbanked. This means they did not have a formal bank account, mainly because they didn't have enough money for the minimum balance required by banks, they didn't trust banks, or there wasn't a bank in close proximity to where they lived. That is one out of four Americans. Still others are underbanked, which means they had a bank account but still used services outside the banking system, such as check cashing and payday loans.

Not having a bank account, or having to pay large fees to cash checks or receive payday loans, severely limits one's ability to save and can lead to long-term debt for borrowers. To help people budget and save, policy change is often required, such as banks not requiring a minimum balance and capping interest fees charged by lenders.

Schedule of SNAP Benefits

Speaking of budgeting and saving money, how often do you get a paycheck? I'm guessing every two weeks. On the other hand, SNAP benefits are allocated once a month. Why do we create an added burden for low-income, food-insecure families to stretch their SNAP dollars throughout an entire month? You've probably heard of the common challenges faced by families receiving SNAP: benefits run out before the end of the month, and that is when people often seek help from food pantries. There is at least anecdotal evidence that some grocery stores raise their prices at the beginning of the month because they know they will have an influx of SNAP customers.

Why not allocate the electronic benefits of SNAP funds twice per month, or even once a week? I understand the historical logic of monthly allocations when food stamps were distributed as paper vouchers in the mail. But now that we have the technology to transfer funds electronically, why can't we flip the switch to add benefits to an account twice monthly? This type of policy change could increase the ability of individuals to budget their monthly finances.

Individual AND Systemic Change

It's important to appreciate the various reasons why individuals may struggle with poverty and food insecurity so we can create holistic solutions. And by understanding the broader systemic reasons why people may become food insecure, we can not only help individuals build skills and social capital but also focus on systems change and advocacy.

"Yes, and," not "either, or." We need both types of approaches. We need individual approaches at the micro-level that can build relationships to foster behavior change, AND we need systems change to reduce barriers to access and mobility at the macro-level.

We want to avoid working only on the extremes:

- Blaming the individual—the person is at fault for their choices and circumstances. If we just teach them how to change their behavior, they will have enough food.
- Blaming the system—the government is to blame. If we simply increase the minimum wage or add money to school systems, we can solve the problem.

A great deal of antipoverty programming and research has been targeted at individuals, with the expectation that if we can teach skills, provide education, and help individuals change their behavior, they will get ahead. These approaches are helpful, but they do not account for the influence of outside factors and structural barriers that work against personal assets. And they often don't consider cultural norms, hidden rules, and mindsets that can keep people set in one economic class. At the same time, waiting for the government or the Gates Foundation to create systems change will overlook many practical steps we can take within our charitable food system.

The following chart outlines different approaches for reducing poverty: working directly with individuals to help them make behavior changes; working with organizations and communities to increase access; and working for systemic and policy change to reduce structural barriers. Each level has value and can play a role in helping people become more food secure, healthy, and financially stable. These are just a few examples.

Levels of Engagement for Poverty Reduction

Level of engagement		
Individuals	Organizations / community	Systems / policy
Budgeting class	Banks that offer no minimum balance for checking accounts; micro-credit or small loans	Earned Income Tax Credit; zoning restrictions for predatory lenders; fair lending practices, such as caps on interest fees allowable
Nutrition education	Nutrition policies at food banks to increase donations of healthy food; improvement of the supply of healthy food at pantries; efforts to make the healthy choice the cheaper and easier choice	Increased Supplemental Nutrition Assistance Program (SNAP) benefits; vouchers for doubling the value of SNAP for purchasing healthy food; funding from the Farm Bill to subsidize diverse fruits and vegetables, not just corn and soybeans
Job training program	Second chance employers who hire people with a criminal record; programs offering transportation services such as Good News Garage or reduced rates for Uber; programs that provide professional attire for those seeking jobs such as Dress for Success	Livable wages; affordable health care and child care; paid sick leave

Find your niche. We need people working on all three levels for individual, organizational, and policy approaches. Where are you called to serve? Do you like working one-on-one with people? Consider providing a class or workshop at the individual level. Maybe you work at an organization and can offer programs or services to help people get ahead. Or perhaps you prefer advocacy and want to influence policy changes at local, state, or federal levels.

You don't have to do this work alone. Join forces with other antipoverty groups who have similar goals but who work in different sectors not related to food. For example,

- Join external advocacy efforts around affordable housing and policies to protect those formerly incarcerated;
- Partner with other state agencies and nonprofit organizations to support the Earned Income Tax Credit and tax preparation assistance; or
- Collaborate with health-care advocates to help enroll people in health insurance plans and health promotion programs.

The Role of Government

It is important to reflect that not long ago, only forty years ago, hunger was seen largely as the federal government's responsibility. Food banks were never expected to provide enough food to solve the problem of hunger. Indeed, food bank directors have argued for years that we cannot "food bank" our way out of hunger.

In response to the challenges created by COVID-19, Feeding America recently stated that "public / private partnerships are critical for the charitable food assistance system. Private industry, non-profit and faith-based organizations and volunteers are needed in tandem with significant government support and cooperation with federal, state and local government agencies."

Think about how many progressive social policies were enacted very quickly with bipartisan support in response to the unprecedented financial impact of COVID-19: providing waivers and flexibility for SNAP applications, increasing SNAP benefits, providing economic stimulus checks, waiving restrictions on school meal distributions, reducing paperwork for government commodity food. As part of the Families First Coronavirus Response Act, certain employers were required to provide paid family and medical leave. Bipartisan policy change is possible. Often Congress will act unanimously during emergencies, such as after 9/11, and then retreat back to their partisan corners. Let this be the watershed moment to realize the immense power of government not only to provide an adequate nutrition safety net but to enact antipoverty policies so that people will not need to rely on government assistance or charitable food.

Advocacy and Policy Change

In order to reduce food insecurity fundamentally, we need to increase our political will to tackle poverty. We need to get in the arena and advocate for policy change. Recognizing that income inequality and systemic injustices create food insecurity can motivate us to advocate for systems change. According to the 2019 USDA Food Security report, states that recently increased their minimum wage (Oregon, Colorado, Nebraska, and New York) had significant drops in food insecurity. Advocating for a livable wage is antihunger work, just as much as distributing pounds of food.

Advocating for a livable wage is antihunger work, just as much as distributing pounds of food.

Closing the Hunger Gap is a network of progressive food organizations, including many food banks, working to expand hunger relief efforts beyond food distribution toward strategies that promote social justice and address the root causes of hunger. WHY Hunger provides resources for creating community solutions focused on equity and justice. Check out their materials and find out who else in your local community is doing antipoverty and antiracism work. Start with your United Way, Habitat for Humanity, and local charitable foundation.

Food banks and food pantries should collaborate with various other social service agencies (such as housing, child welfare, transportation, and health care) because we're fighting for the same supports and for the same people. Our voices are stronger together.

Action Steps

- Talk about structural racism and injustices across racial, gender, and class lines. Start the conversation with your staff, volunteers, and local partners.
- Check out the ALICE project by United Way. Share resources with your staff and other community partners to advocate for better income supports for those working low-wage jobs.
- Read about the Bridges Out of Poverty framework and hold discussions in your organization and with community partners to create a shared language about class and ways to build bridges.
- Ask politicians running for office for their stance on hunger and how they will address it.
- Think about when your programs are open. Is it Monday through Friday during work hours? Consider opening on some evenings and weekends to accommodate working families.
- Pay livable wages at your place of employment. Advocate for livable wages at local, state, and federal levels.
- Consider offering the Bridges Out of Poverty workshop or Getting Ahead classes as part of your programming. Talk with a local business or foundation to support the costs.

As Martin Luther King Jr. said, "You don't have to see the whole staircase, just take the first step."

Resources

Alexander, Michelle. *The New Jim Crow: Mass Incarceration in the Age of Color-blindness*. New York: The New Press, 2012.

DiAngelo, Robin. *White Fragility: Why It's So Hard for White People to Talk About Racism*. Boston: Beacon Press, 2018.

Jindra, Michael, and Ines W. Jindra. "Poverty and the Controversial Work of Nonprofits." *Social Science and Public Policy* 53 (2016): 634–640. https://www.academia.edu/29592004/Poverty_and_the_Controversial_Work_of_Nonprofits.

Kendi, Ibram X. *How to Be an Anti-Racist*. New York: One World, 2019.

Neighborhood Trust Financial Partners. https://www.neighborhoodtrust.org/.

Payne, Ruby K., Philip E. DeVol, and Terie Dreussi Smith. *Bridges Out of Poverty: Strategies for Professionals and Communities*. aha! Process. https://www.ahaprocess.com/bridges-out-of-poverty-strategies-for-professionals-and-communities/.

United Way. "United for ALICE." https://www.unitedforalice.org/overview.

Vance, J. D. *Hillbilly Elegy: A Memoir of a Family and Culture in Crisis*. New York: Harper Collins Publishers, 2016.

WHY Hunger. https://whyhunger.org/.

CHAPTER 11

Equity within Food Banks and Pantries

A few years ago when I was visiting a food bank, a staff member was giving me a tour of their facility when she made a comment about the carpet versus the concrete. I didn't know what she meant so I asked her to explain. She described what I have come to realize is a common divide within food banks. The warehouse staff, who are usually in lower-paid positions and blue-collar jobs, work on concrete floors, whereas those with higher-paid positions, the executive team and white-collar jobs, have offices with carpet. Sometimes this is described as the downstairs (warehouse) versus upstairs (executive offices). Rather than viewing this as simply an accurate description of our organizational chart, we can recognize inequalities within our organizations and use that recognition as an opportunity to build more equity. For example, we can ensure that frontline workers have a voice at the table when programmatic decisions are being made. We can solicit input from staff throughout the organization to show we value their opinion.

If we want to reduce structural inequalities and build equity in our communities through external advocacy, we should also examine how we live our values internally, in our organizations. This chapter will focus on ways to involve the people we serve, to hear their voices and concerns, and use their input to design our programs and services. Let's start by discussing ways that food banks can promote equity from within, to create bridges between the carpet and concrete.

Equity in Our Workplace

Many organizations are striving to become more diverse, equitable, and inclusive. At Foodshare, two years ago we hosted a diversity training to help us on this journey. All staff spent half a day in the boardroom as we discussed difficult topics of race and class. It flopped. It did not have the desired effect, and staff members felt like it was a waste of time. The facilitators meant well, but rather than bringing us together as a group, several staff members felt more divided and uncomfortable after the training. The conversations seemed to highlight differences rather than common ground.

But we didn't give up. We failed forward and tried to learn from what didn't work. Last year we hired a different consulting group and held a second training for all staff to explore ways that race, class, gender identity, and privilege impact us personally and ways that we as an organization can cultivate a culture of inclusion in which diverse perspectives are valued. The training went well. As we discussed in the last chapter, talking about these issues is challenging, but it can also make us stronger and more compassionate.

In 2019 Foodshare created a staff-led Equity, Diversity and Inclusion (EDI) committee with a bottom-up approach to discussing diversity issues rather than a top-down decision coming from the board of directors. One of the tasks of the committee was to revise Foodshare's EDI policy. The committee members discussed the goals of the policy, and it went through several iterations before it was presented to the leadership

We recognize that systemic injustices—such as racism, classism, and sexism—create and perpetuate conditions that sustain poverty and hunger.

team and then finally to the board of directors. The recently approved EDI policy reads: "Our Vision includes magnifying the voices of people who have experienced hunger and welcoming diverse perspectives. To live these ideals every day, we foster and promote a workplace where all cultures, faiths, ethnicities, and individual differences are welcome. We strive for equity and a work environment that welcomes everyone's perspective and contribution. We recognize that systemic injustices—such as racism, classism, and sexism—create and perpetuate conditions that sustain poverty and hunger. Foodshare believes that all voices have the right to be heard in an environment of equity, respect, and inclusion."

The EDI committee also coordinates "lunch and learn" sessions to have informal conversations about diversity and to create a safe space for people to talk about their lived experiences. Edna Bailey, the volunteer services manager at Foodshare, shared her experience of growing up in poverty with staff at a recent lunch. She said, "My environment growing up, we were poor and I didn't realize we were poor. But I never went to bed hungry. If you haven't lived it you don't know. Even if you have lived it, your experience won't be the same. Your definition of being poor won't be the same." She cautioned about passing judgment and making assumptions about others, both in the office and in the community.

Edna described how she has heard comments from staff or volunteers that work at food distributions about who is deserving of food. For example, "If we see a family coming to a Mobile program and they look a certain way, then they need it (the food). But if they look another way, then staff or volunteers will question whether they need it." You never know what another person's experience has been or what brings them to the food pantry line. She encouraged staff not to make assumptions and not to judge.

Along with examining our own attitudes, we can improve our workplace practices, including how much we pay our workers. In 2018, Foodshare increased our minimum hourly wage to $15. But Connecticut has a high cost of living, so we realize that it can be difficult to make ends meet even making $15 an hour. Our mission statement is to lead an informed, coordinated response to hunger in our community. We shouldn't assume that hunger is elsewhere. We can start from within. We designed a confidential program in which staff can go to the human resources office if they have trouble getting enough food, and they will receive a gift card to a local grocery store. A few staff members now request help monthly.

Leadership and Decision Making

Often, the boardrooms of food banks are filled with executives from local businesses. These individuals bring tremendous talent and business savvy to the table. They are incredibly generous with their time. And there is an expectation that they will also be generous with donations to the food bank. It can be equally important to include members of our food pantry network at the table as well, those with firsthand and real-world experience addressing the problem of hunger, even if they are not able to make a large financial donation.

At the Oregon Food Bank, staff incorporate ways to build equity throughout their organization, including their mission statement, having food pantry staff or clients on their board of directors, and putting clients in the center of their work. Every other year they conduct a five-question survey with board members about experiences with hunger. They ask whether members have ever used a food pantry, received free or reduced school meals, or used SNAP. Susannah Morgan, CEO of the Oregon Food Bank, says that they find ways for people to speak about their experiences with hunger during board meetings.

Susannah described how the Oregon legislature was considering a statewide mandate to set a cap of 7 percent for the maximum amount landlords could raise rents. Like most places around the country, high housing costs were the single biggest driver to needing food assistance in Oregon. The food bank was thinking about taking a position on the mandate and discussed it at a board meeting. A board member, who is a renter and tenant, spoke passionately about the burden of rent and how much it drove her economic choices. She also spoke from the perspective of an African American woman. She described how African American women are vastly overrepresented among renters, largely because of systemic inequalities and disadvantages for building wealth. The fact that she was able to bring her identities to the board meeting changed the course of the discussion. Without her voice and lived experience, the conversation might have gone in a different direction. The board and Oregon Food Bank supported the legislation, which then passed.

Similarly, when major decisions are being made about food bank programs, it's critical to hear from people who will use the program. Input is extremely helpful on issues such as where the program will be located, when the program will operate, what to call the new program, and how to promote it in the community. Enlisting participant perspectives may mean that it takes longer to design and launch the program, but it will be more likely to be accepted and sustained in the community when there is buy-in and engagement from those who will benefit. This is a way to diversify power when making decisions and to provide greater community representation.

Reinventing our charitable food system and shifting the paradigm for how our organizations operate requires strong leaders. Jason Jakubowski, the president and CEO of Foodshare, is not only a strong leader himself, he has dramatically changed the power dynamics and circle of leadership throughout our organization. In his three years at Foodshare, he has broadened the leadership team by about 500 percent. Historically, key decisions were made by the top three officials within the organization, with limited input from other staff members. Now we fill our boardroom for monthly leadership meetings with over twenty people who provide input and help make decisions. Jason empowers staff to see themselves as leaders and recognizes leadership in every department, from the carpet to the concrete. He also recruited a new cohort of board members to increase diversity, including a member from a local community college and from a housing authority that run partner programs within our network.

The Need to Feel Seen

Have you ever noticed when you go to a sporting event, especially a baseball game, that when the camera crew broadcasts someone's image on the jumbotron screen, the person becomes ecstatic? They grin ear to ear, they wave enthusiastically, sometimes they get up and do a dance. Why? Because they see themselves on the big screen. It doesn't matter that it's in front of thousands of other people. There they are, larger than life, and they love it!

We all like to be seen. To be heard. This matters for our work in charitable food because often the people we serve are not represented.

We all like to be seen. To be heard. This matters for our work in charitable food because often the people we serve are not represented. Think about the key decision makers at your food bank or your food pantry. Do they represent the demographics of your community? Have any of them experienced food insecurity? Making sure that diverse voices and experiences are informing important decisions in our organizations is a powerful step to creating more equity and inclusion. This can include representation on the board of directors, but it can also mean asking the people we serve for their opinions to help inform our work.

When there is a race, class, or power divide between those receiving food and those providing food, it is more likely that voices will be silenced. We discussed this with the role of volunteers and traditional food pantries that don't offer choice. As we design pantries to provide full choice, and space for people to interact, we create opportunities to listen and to share stories. Just as people like to see their faces on the screen at a ballgame, people want to know that their opinion matters.

My colleagues at Urban Alliance in East Hartford, Connecticut, have a thoughtful way of capturing the faces and voices of the people who participate in their programs. Urban Alliance's goal is to create opportunities for people to achieve lasting change in their lives through the collaborative work of churches and organizations in the local community. They build capacity to reduce poverty. When you walk into their office, they have huge displays of colorful pictures and quotes from people who participate in their various initiatives. They don't show downtrodden images of people struggling; they capture the hope and vibrancy of people who are working toward goals and self-sufficiency. When you look at the beautiful photographs, you can almost picture the images on a big jumbotron screen.

The Importance of Individuals' Stories

One of Foodshare's three-year strategic priorities is to raise awareness about hunger. One way to do this is to amplify the voices of those who have experienced food insecurity, poverty, and injustice. To help achieve this goal, I encouraged our communications team and other staff members to gather stories from the people we serve, to ask their permission to share their stories, to take photographs, and to include these stories from real people in our network who benefit from our services. I described Ethical Storytelling, which according to the website is "a way of stewarding the stories of others, to listen to the voice of the constituent as our teacher, to offer a diversity of voices, experiences and opinions, and to take a posture of learning."

Too often the way we raise awareness about hunger is through national statistics about the millions of people who are food insecure and the millions of pounds of food we distributed. It's hard to wrap your head around what this means for a family. My colleague Andrew Janavey is the digital media specialist at Foodshare, and not only is he a talented photographer and designer, he really gets it. He understands the value of putting the people we serve in the center of what we do.

> *Too often the way we raise awareness about hunger is through national statistics about the millions of people who are food insecure and the millions of pounds of food we distributed. It's hard to wrap your head around what this means for a family.*

Andrew describes how "food banks work on staggering scales . . . hundreds of thousands of people, millions of meals, etc. And while these numbers are certainly awe inspiring, I think some of our true impact is lost on the public when we primarily communicate in this way. Most people probably don't have any idea how many pounds of food the average person eats in a month or how many people live in their county so these big numbers become nothing more than just that . . . big numbers. This is where the individual stories of our clients can help communicate that true impact."

Andrew started visiting some of our local agencies with our partner program staff and has been incorporating ethical storytelling into his work, sharing quotes and beautiful photos of people who benefit from our programs. He describes how "a hundred thousand struggling people and tens of thousands of struggling children is difficult to imagine, but an evicted mother cooking ravioli for kids in a motel room coffee maker is not. That's why story collection is important for me, because what we do is more than just the total sum of all the numbers. There are real people at every step of the process. On a personal level, interacting directly with clients recharges my passion for my work."

For food bank staff who already interact with clients and partner agencies, you can encourage them to gather quotes and share stories as a natural, comfortable part of their job. You can then share these stories in your communications to describe the diverse ways that hunger impacts your community. Ideally, this is a three-way street (I know, that may cause a traffic jam, but bear with me). We gather stories to listen to and empower those who experience hunger so they feel seen and heard. At the same time, by listening to their experiences, we gain a better appreciation for their situation, which will help us as we design programs and will improve our ability to advocate for and with others. And by sharing their stories and experiences, we can raise awareness of the impact of hunger locally with donors and supporters.

People may have heard of a local food bank or food pantry, but they often don't really know what we do. At a drive-through food distribution during COVID-19, Geri from Ellington, Connecticut, was picking up food for her family and she said, "I have donated to Foodshare in the past. I knew it helped people but I didn't know how it helped until I went through it myself." Sharing stories will help others have a better appreciation for the impact of our work and the people we serve.

So much of the communications, websites, and social media from food banks highlight pallets of food, large check presentations from corporations, and pictures of volunteers sorting food, with little mention of the people we are serving. Andrew Janavey says that "it's rare to come across a photo of what happens to any of it in the end. If we do show a food distribution it's often from across a parking lot. If we do show a client, they're often being handed food." Ethical story gathering and storytelling is an important step to raise awareness among staff, donors, and volunteers about hunger and to engage the people we serve to tell their own story.

Ethical Storytelling

When we create opportunities for staff, volunteers, and food pantry guests to interact, moving from transactional to relational, we will engage in more conversations. This may be with a designated greeter at a food pantry, a co-shopper in a client choice pantry, in a waiting area where guests sit before they collect their food, or in workshops or focus groups to gather feedback. The process of gathering qualitative data should be informal and conversational, not intimidating (both for staff and clients). When you hear an important comment or someone describing how hunger impacts them or how the food pantry has helped them, ask if the person would be willing to share their story. Many people want to be heard and recognized. They want to be on the jumbotron camera. Asking to share their story can be empowering for people who may often feel invisible or silenced.

Here are some basic steps for gathering and sharing stories ethically, to respect the dignity of those we serve. Remember, it starts with creating space and time to have conversations and listen to the people that we serve.

1. As part of your conversation, ask if you can take down a quote on paper or a smart phone.
2. Read the quote back, ask if you captured it right and if there is anything else they want to share.

3. Ask for permission to share the quote anonymously, with a name, or by town.
4. You can ask if they would like their photo taken with the quote.
5. You can use a media consent form to receive formal permission to use the quote or photograph.

Describe why we want to share their story: to help people understand how hunger impacts our communities; so others who experience hunger won't feel alone; and to reduce stereotypes about who experiences hunger and why. We can help raise awareness about how food banks help people, not just through the number of pounds we distribute, but by sharing stories from people who have received the food to describe the impact it makes on their lives.

Opportunities to Build Social Capital

Sharing quotes and photos is a first step in engaging people in your work. Creating space and opportunity for people to meet, interact, and build relationships is a larger step for more transformational change. In his book *Bowling Alone*, Robert Putnam describes how "your economic opportunities are affected not just by who you are, but by who your neighbors are and how well you know them. 'Networking' works, so frayed networks mean more poverty." Rather than simply being places where people come to get food, food pantries can be designed as community hubs where people network, particularly across race and class lines. We can build a sense of community within food pantries, creating space for interactions.

We are all familiar with social support, or bonding capital, which you receive from people in your inner circle of family and friends. These are people that are very much like you. Bridging capital is the type of social support you receive from people outside your social circle, from

people who may not have a lot in common with you. These less familiar connections can lead to job opportunities, networking, and other
opportunities to get ahead.

I'm sure you've heard of the golden rule—treat others the way you
want to be treated. I would encourage you, whenever possible, to use
the platinum rule—treat others the way they want to be treated. How
will we know how they want to be treated? Ask them, spend time with
them, and build relationships.

An example of building social capital is
through the Circles USA program in which
middle-income and high-income volunteers,
or "allies," meet with people in poverty to
support them and help them navigate ways
to reduce poverty. Who you know matters.
The Circles program collects data when participants start the program and then every six
months during the program. They document
results for individuals and also for communities. Their results show that participants
have increased income, less dependence on
public assistance, and expanded support networks. Communities that
use the Circles USA program have changed attitudes about poverty and
have influenced policy changes.

I would encourage you, whenever possible, to use the platinum rule—treat others the way they want to be treated. How will we know how they want to be treated? Ask them, spend time with them, and build relationships.

When individuals participate in the Getting Ahead program or Circles program, it creates space to share community-level issues that make
it hard to get enough food. People share insights about the effect of low
wages, negligent landlords, lack of transportation, grocery stores that
charge more at the beginning of the month, and so on. Clients can
serve as powerful advocates for policy change. Food pantries can provide
opportunities to explore these systemic issues and to raise the voices of
those impacted. Now we're talking about transformational change.

Advocacy

One of the goals from the national Closing the Hunger Gap network is to "support grassroots movements led by the people most impacted by the root causes of poverty and hunger." To take another step toward equity and inclusion, food banks and food pantries can partner with local organizations that focus on advocacy, community organizing, and social justice. Here are a few great examples.

Witnesses to Hunger was started in Philadelphia in 2008 and has several local chapters, including in New Haven, Connecticut. Witnesses are a group of experts on hunger, those who have experienced food insecurity and poverty, and who advocate for policy changes at the local, state, and national levels. Their mission is to unite the community by sharing stories of their lived experiences, educating community members and policy makers, and advocating for social and economic justice.

The Open Door Food Shelf in Minnesota created a program called the Leadership Table as a way to involve and empower their food shelf users. The program provides stipends for clients to discuss food security issues, builds public speaking skills about how to use one's voice for social justice and how to talk with legislators, and provides opportunities for clients to share their experiences with local decision makers. The program is not simply about hearing the voices of participants but about empowering clients to advocate for themselves and their community.

According to Sarah Kinney from Partnership for a Healthier America, who spent years working with food shelves in Minnesota, Open Door invited members of the Leadership Table to a Food Justice Summit. The food shelf recognized the value of the advocates to share their stories and provided the resources to enable them to attend the summit. The clients received free registration, hotel, meals and transportation. They went to the summit with food shelf staff to share their views and to hear the bigger conversation about food security.

Levels of Public Participation

You may have figured out by this point in the book that I like the idea of spectrums and continuums. I rarely see things as black or white, yes or no, all or nothing. This book creates a big vision and roadmap for where we want to go as a charitable food system, but I don't want you to get intimidated by thinking you have to go from zero to sixty all at once. Taking incremental steps is far better than sticking with the status quo. Feeding America describes these steps as "on-ramps," different strategies to help people and organizations get on the road and start driving toward change.

Here are examples of steps to build equity, involve diverse groups from your community, and include people who have experienced hunger. The categories below are part of the spectrum of public participation and describe opportunities to involve the people you serve, from low to high involvement:

- Inform—provide information on your website, in newsletters, and in fundraising appeals to describe the problem of hunger in your community and how your food bank or food pantry is addressing it. This involves little to no input from the public.
- Consult—gather feedback and opinions about the problem of hunger or about services you provide. Start by listening to the public through focus groups, surveys, or interviews.
- Involve—work directly with the public as you design and develop programs to ensure that different voices are heard and considered. If you have guests who are already engaged as volunteers in your organization, they can become involved with making decisions, providing feedback, and helping to design programs.
- Collaborate—partner with the public through advisory committees in each step of the process to develop solutions. Elicit public input

and advice about the decisions you make. Involve other antipoverty and social justice organizations to partner with you as you design and launch a new program. Include community partners in grant proposals to create shared ownership.

- Empower—implement programs that were designed by the public. Local community members, particularly people who have experienced hunger, should make the final decisions about programming or services.

Best Practices for Engaging People with Lived Experience

Rather than hosting training meetings at the food bank, consider hosting meetings at community locations and use it as an opportunity to highlight superstar programs in your network.

Here are some suggestions for ways to increase equity and inclusion in food banks and food pantries. Host accessible meetings and programs—consider what days and times will be most convenient for those you are trying to help. Consider providing day care, a meal, and possibly transportation to include people with lived experience. Rather than hosting training meetings at the food bank, consider hosting meetings at community locations and use it as an opportunity to highlight superstar programs in your network. Make sure that people who are marginalized feel welcome to participate. For example, the LGBTQ (lesbian, gay, bisexual, transgender, queer) population may not feel welcome attending programs at a church. Make sure the location is accessible for people with disabilities.

Consider paying people with lived experience for their time. If you want to gather input through focus groups or surveys, provide incentives such as gift cards or cash. The Getting Ahead program provides stipends each week for the investigators as part of their program to recognize the value of their time. I know you're probably working with a limited budget. Get creative. Ask a local company to donate gift cards or a small piece of merchandise. This is also a great opportunity to raise awareness about your programs with local companies so they learn about how you are offering services beyond food.

Take the time to build trust. When we move from trying to move food as efficiently as possible to building relationships and trust, it is important to recognize that this will take more time. Build in additional time to meet and greet people that you serve. Set realistic expectations about starting a new program that includes feedback from those you want to serve. Talk with your donors about the added benefits you hope to achieve but also the additional time and resources this will take.

Diversify representation and deepen engagement. Think about the diversity of people who are involved as staff, volunteers, and board members in your organization. Include more diverse viewpoints and experiences to engage people from different socioeconomic classes. As you hold meetings, look around the table and think about who is missing. Invite new faces and new perspectives to your next meeting. And if this is challenging, go back to the first suggestion to make sure your meetings are in accessible locations and at convenient times.

As you think about these different levels of engagement, keep in mind: the faster we go, the more we will inform and exclude the people we are serving. To co-design programs and include other community groups in the decision-making process requires time, trust, and relationships. We need to slow down and take considerably more time to be inclusive and to empower people in our community to be advocates for their behalf. A common theme throughout this book is that efficiency can sometimes detract us from effectiveness. As the African proverb says, "If you want to go fast, go alone. If you want to go far, go together."

Action Steps

- Ask your guests for their input and opinion. Start the conversation with a sense of curiosity, describe how you want to learn and understand their perspective. Go into the conversation suspending the belief that you are the expert on the situation.
- Create an organizational value of hearing and including the voices of people who experience hunger and make sure this value is upheld by staff members.
- Use ethical storytelling to listen to the people you serve and ask their permission to share their lived experiences with food insecurity. Show their strengths and goals through their quotes and in photos.
- Create an equity, diversity, and inclusion policy for your organization or set up a committee of diverse members to discuss these issues.
- Include a member of a food pantry on the board of your food bank, or a client as a board member of your food pantry.
- Be a leader. Make one change.

Resources

Circles USA. https://www.circlesusa.org/.

Closing the Hunger Gap. https://thehungergap.org/.

Ethical Storytelling. www.ethicalstorytelling.com.

Homer, Alison. *Engaging People with Lived/Living Experience: A Guide for Including People in Poverty Reduction*. Tamarack Institute, 2019. https://www.tamarack community.ca/hubfs/Resources/Publications/10-Engaging%20People%20 With%20LivedLiving%20Experience%20of%20Poverty.pdf.

Saul, Nick, and Andrea Curtis. *The Stop: How the Fight for Good Food Transformed a Community and Inspired a Movement*. Brooklyn, NY: Melville House, 2013.

The Open Door. "The Open Door Pantry Leadership Table." https://theopendoor
pantry.org/the-open-door-leadership-table/.

"What Is the Spectrum of Public Participation?" *Sustaining Community: Families,
Community, the Environment (blog)*. https://sustainingcommunity.wordpress
.com/2017/02/14/spectrum-of-public-participation/.

CHAPTER 12

New Partners and Community Food Hubs

This is a particularly exciting time in the charitable food system because new organizations are interested in partnering with food banks and food pantries. Hospitals, clinics, colleges, and universities are recognizing that their patients and students are often food insecure, and they are finding creative ways to tackle hunger. These are great opportunities to use best practices right from the beginning when new initiatives are being established. I hope this book can be a helpful guide for new organizations that are just getting started and may not have thought about how to design or run a food pantry.

This chapter starts with some opportunities for partnering with new organizations in your community and other ways to serve people in convenient locations to meet people where they are. Then it focuses on existing food pantry networks. I describe a rationale and make suggestions for consolidating some existing food pantries to provide a more coordinated approach to hunger. We finish with a vision for a comprehensive network of community food hubs that provide food and much more. We can't tackle hunger alone, and we will be stronger when we work with others. New partners can also bring new ideas and fresh perspectives to help us question the status quo.

Food as Medicine

In 2018, the United States spent about $3.6 trillion on health care. Did you notice the *t*? Yes, that was trillions. We spend substantially more on health care than other high-income countries, and yet we are sicker and have worse health outcomes. In an effort to reduce the costs of health care and to reduce health disparities, health-care providers and insurance companies are focusing on the underlying risk factors that contribute to poor health, including the social determinants of health. Research has shown that not having enough food and not being able to afford and access healthy, nutritious food contributes to poor health.

Many health-care providers are beginning to address food insecurity, which starts by identifying who is food insecure. Many hospitals and health clinics are beginning to ask patients about food insecurity using the two-item Hunger Vital Sign questions that I described in chapter 9. When patients screen positive for being food insecure, the clinicians have a variety of ways that they can intervene. Medical staff can refer food insecure patients to local food pantries or provide information about enrolling in the SNAP program. Some clinics provide a prescription to a food pantry on-site to make it super convenient for patients to get extra food. When the doctor recognizes that a patient is food insecure, the doctor can refer the patient to a healthy food pantry where they can select nutritious food before they leave the clinic or hospital.

The Fresh Food Farmacy was created in 2016 by Geisinger Health in central Pennsylvania as a model program that has received national attention. The comprehensive program helps reduce obesity and diabetes while increasing food security. The program identifies patients with type 2 diabetes who are food insecure and works in collaboration with doctors, nurses, pharmacists, dieticians, a wellness team, and food pantry staff to offer diabetes education with a health coach and nutritional counseling. The program also partners with the Central Pennsylvania Food Bank to provide ten meals per week of diabetes appropriate food.

More than six hundred individuals have participated in the Fresh Food Farmacy, and Geisinger reports some pretty terrific results. Patients have significant reductions in their blood sugar levels (HbA1c) and are better able to manage their diabetes with fewer complications. Patients report exercising more, quitting smoking, and feeling more confident in their ability to manage chronic diseases.

Another great example of providing food as medicine is the Preventive Food Pantry at Boston Medical Center, which opened in 2011. Primary care doctors identify low-income patients at risk for food insecurity and chronic diseases and provide a prescription to visit the food pantry up to twice per month. The manager of the Preventive Food Pantry is a registered dietetic technician who can determine what foods are appropriate for a patient's dietary needs, as prescribed by the physician. Pantry staff includes members who are fluent in four different languages, which increases accessibility.

In order to be successful, we want to enable clinicians to adequately screen and also know how to intervene.

But here's a catch. While the two-question Hunger Vital Sign is a simple and quick tool to identify if patients are food insecure, some clinicians are asking the two questions but don't know what to tell patients for referrals. Other clinicians choose not to ask the questions because they don't know what services or programs are available to treat food insecurity. Let's help connect the dots. There is a great opportunity for food banks to collaborate with local health-care providers to provide information about available food pantries and SNAP outreach. In order to be successful, we want to enable clinicians to adequately screen and also know how to intervene.

Like any type of relationship, it can take time to build partnerships between food banks or pantries and health-care providers. You need to take time to first understand each other. Kim Prendergast, who worked at Feeding America and now works at Community Care Cooperative (C3) in Massachusetts, says, "What makes sense if you're partnering with a hospital is different than a health insurance company. Understanding the unique challenges and the sand box in which they are playing, is really important." For example, groups may seem to speak a different language, so you need to take time to get on the same page. Social determinants of health (SDOH) and EPIC (a platform for electronic medical records) may be new terms for a food bank.

Take time to discuss the goals and time lines of different partners to make sure you have a mutual understanding of what a potential partnership involves. Codesigning a program, like a food pantry within a hospital or clinic, takes more time and trust. But it is more likely to be sustainable than if one group designs the program without feedback from the other.

Food pantries can be ideal sites for health promotion and disease prevention. Nursing students, nutrition educators, and clinical staff can meet with clients who are at risk for diabetes, hypertension, and other chronic diseases and provide blood pressure and blood glucose screening, testing, and/or monitoring. Partnerships between food banks or food pantries and health-care providers is a promising field with a lot of room for growth. Some potential partners include the Root Cause Coalition, Hunger 2 Health Collaboratory, ProMedica, Federally Qualified Health Centers, and Kaiser Permanente, as well as other health insurance companies. If you haven't already, start building relationships with health-care providers in your area to start offering food as medicine.

College Hunger

The stereotypical image of a college student is a privileged young adult who goes to school full-time for four years and whose parents pay for all expenses. But today the reality is quite different for many students. The makeup of college students has changed dramatically over the past two decades, with more diversity and more nontraditional students over age twenty-five. The costs of tuition, room, and board have skyrocketed well beyond the rates of inflation. More than half of college students need some type of financial assistance.

Many college students are under tremendous financial pressure to pay for the costs associated with college and may not be able to afford food. In response, colleges and universities are finding creative ways to address food insecurity on campus. With funding from The Kresge Foundation and in collaboration with Claremont Graduate University, in 2019 Feeding America released a report about college hunger. They conducted a survey of the 200 food banks in Feeding America's network, and 150 responded. They found that 110 food banks do some type of direct food distribution, including food pantries on campuses and mobile food distributions; 39 food banks help college students apply for SNAP; and 33 food banks are involved in advocacy efforts related to college hunger.

Ways to Address Hunger on Campus

One approach is to identify students who are food insecure and provide extra meals through the traditional student meal plan.

Just as the Feeding America study found, there are various ways to address hunger on college campuses. One approach is to identify students who are food insecure and provide extra meals through the traditional student meal plan. Just like SNAP dollars allow people to shop for food at the grocery store, this approach allows students to eat meals on campus with their peers.

Monica Sager is a rising senior at Clark University and an ambassador for the Campus Hunger Project with Challah for Hunger, a national program that supports college students to develop solutions to hunger. Monica has created a program to tackle student hunger that will be anonymous and without stigma. Through her plan, the financial aid office will identify students in need, because students are already reporting their financial information, and the business office will add money to the "one card," which is used in the dining hall or for to-go meals on campus. The business office will add five meals per week throughout the school year for students in need. The project will be funded by the student government, and the university president has agreed to double the funding. Monica's initiative is similar to the Swipe Out Hunger program where college students can donate unused meals from their meal plan to help support other students struggling with food insecurity.

But what about campuses that don't have dining halls, such as community colleges, or for commuter students that don't eat meals on campus? Designing a food pantry on campus can be a different approach. Ideally, you want to avoid a pantry that will cause a lot of stigma by identifying students as poor. Think about the other best practices I've been preaching about throughout this book. Design a pantry with client choice, providing wraparound services such as SNAP outreach and wellness programs, and create a welcoming space. You get it.

Asnuntuck Community College in Enfield, Connecticut, recognized that many students were struggling with food insecurity, and so they created a food pantry. It was in a small room the size of a janitor's office. They had a few committed students and staff running the pantry, but trust me, it wasn't pretty. The pantry director applied for a small grant from Foodshare to improve their pantry. In 2019 they moved to a space eight times the size of the original pantry and now provide food and much more. The pantry is bright and welcoming and is staffed by students. The pantry is designed as fully client choice, promoting healthy food with the SWAP stoplight system, and they also include personal hygiene items. There is a wellness space where professionals help students apply for health insurance and other community services and where students can relax. The pantry is designed to promote a sense of self-worth and accomplishment and to foster a sense of fellowship and belonging.

Sherry Paquette is the director of the Cougar Pantry (the name comes from the school mascot at Asnuntuck Community College). She said, "We see Foodshare not as a place just to pick up food, but as a true partner. With the grant that we got [from Foodshare], we were able to purchase a double wide glass front refrigerator and a stand up freezer which enabled us to increase our abundance of healthy food options. Now we can take in more dairy, more fruits, tons of vegetables, and we can help our students to lead a healthier lifestyle."

Foodshare staff recently asked our partner programs to share success stories from clients using their programs. Here are a few examples from the Asnuntuck Community College that illustrate the reality of being food insecure yet striving for a better life:

- "One young man was living in a tent on a friend's property last spring. He told me at the time that the Pantry was keeping him alive. He is adamant that he will stay in college and graduate. He still uses the Pantry and volunteers his time there. He is now staying with another student and just got a part time job."
- "A single mom going to school here has her child in the free daycare program on campus for when she is in class. She uses the Pantry to keep her and her child fed. She is struggling to work two part time jobs and go to school while keeping a roof over her child. She is desperate to improve her life and be a role model for her child. She hugs me all the time and says thanks for the Pantry."
- "I could go on for days—I could literally give you 20–30 success stories without blinking an eye. Our students are choosing between food and books, food and gas for their vehicles if they even have a

vehicle. Many have no primary healthcare provider and have no way to pay for medical attention or medicine if they are sick. However—they are literally changing their own lives by getting an education."

Success stories similar to those at Asnuntuck Community College can be found around the country. As people have become aware of food insecurity among college students, on-campus pantries have become very popular. Yet it's important to consider the resources you have available within a college or university to address food insecurity. If there is limited space for a food pantry, limited people power to staff it, and limited refrigeration so you'll need to provide only nonperishable food, does a food pantry really make sense? Would it be better to allocate resources for meal swipes or gift cards to local grocery stores for students in need?

There are a wide variety of projects addressing food insecurity on college campuses. Monica Sager says, "It's important to recognize that there won't be one big solution" to hunger. This is true for college campuses but also in other programs throughout our communities. You want to determine what makes sense for your local situation and with the resources that you have available.

New Partners

I've highlighted health-care providers and college campuses as new anti-hunger partners. Food banks can help identify other populations at high risk of food insecurity, such as children, and devise innovative solutions to meet people where they already are working, learning, playing, and shopping. Can you partner with community service organizations, libraries, YMCAs, Boys & Girls Clubs, schools, or recreation centers? Think of strong anchor organizations in your community and ways to create one-stop shopping opportunities to address hunger. Get creative.

When you are designing a new food pantry, you have an opportunity to utilize all the tools we've been discussing in this book. When an organization wants to start a food pantry, invite them to visit some of the stellar pantries in the area so they can see a model program. It may not always make sense to create a stand-alone food pantry or community kitchen. It might be better to offer a healthy mobile program where the food bank provides free food to a community site on a regular schedule or to engage in SNAP outreach.

Colleges and universities can also be valuable partners that can help with programming and evaluation of the work you're doing. Reach out to a local college or university to see if student interns are available. Nursing students can provide health screenings, nutrition students can provide education and help rank food with the SWAP stoplight system, social work students can support coaches that provide case management and referrals. Reach out to faculty members who may be looking for community-based projects and could help conduct research to evaluate the work you are doing. Funders like to see outcomes, so these research partnerships can help garner new funding.

Approaches to Serving Excluded Groups

In every state and most every community, there are demographic pockets of people who are underserved because they are not part of the mainstream, dominant population. Their voices are often not heard, their input not included in decision making. Start by identifying groups that may be excluded, thinking about race, gender identity, language, sexual orientation, or legal status. How do we create programs by, for, and with them? We will likely need new partners and allies to reach new populations.

For example, the Oregon Food Bank recognized that many in the LGBTQ (lesbian, gay, bisexual, transgender, queer) community felt very uncomfortable going to churches, where food programs are often located. Once the food bank identified the problem, it provided trainings for how organizations could create a safe space and developed an LGBTQ affirming group of programs, including some churches. The food bank provides a listing of LGBTQ affirming agencies to the public, and the agencies display a window decal with a rainbow design to highlight their designation.

Start by identifying groups that may be excluded, thinking about race, gender identity, language, sexual orientation, or legal status. How do we create programs by, for, and with them?

Think about disenfranchised groups such as immigrants without legal status. When food programs have long lines of customers, the agency may enlist the help of local police for crowd control. This may not be a welcoming scene for someone who doesn't have legal status, and they may not feel comfortable going to get food. This is another great reason to find ways to reduce the wait time and the need to have lines of people that require policing.

Language barriers can be a challenge for new immigrants. Can you partner with a local refugee program, Catholic Charities, or other social service program that is an entry point in the community? Can you work with a local translation service to make sure your program materials are in the languages spoken in your community? Find a client who speaks the language who can help translate materials and communicate with peers about the program and services that are available (and pay them for their time). This could also be a good opportunity to partner with a community group that can provide an English as a Second Language class at your agency.

In addition to working with new partners like health clinics and colleges, much work can be done within our existing food pantry networks. Food banks can help determine where gaps exist, where food insecurity is greatest, and where there are potential duplications of services. And this can lead to the vision of creating community food hubs. So let's explore how we get there.

Succession Planning and New Leadership

Because most food pantries were established during the 1980s and 1990s, there is a generation of food pantry directors who are nearing retirement. Who will take their place? If you are involved with a food pantry, is there a plan for when the director retires? Who will step in? If we want to ensure that we are serving our communities well, it's important to take some time to plan for what's next. Ideally, you can meet with other food pantries and social service agencies in your community to strategize and collaborate about next steps. Perhaps this is a good time to merge with another pantry. Food banks can serve a leadership role and help with this process by routinely asking their network of programs if they have a succession plan and if they would consider merging with another program.

Who can serve as new leaders to help run food pantries? How do we motivate young adults to become engaged in food banks and food pantries? When food banks are hiring, how do we recruit college graduates? I'm encouraged by college students who are majoring in food systems and food justice. There is an opportunity for these students who have been grounded in social justice classes, and who may have experienced food insecurity themselves, to help reinvent the way we address hunger. Imagine if food banks, food pantries, and new antihunger programs hire young leaders who are passionate about food justice. What will this system look like?

Most young adults are idealistic and want to change the world. If we describe a food pantry position, whether paid or volunteer, as simply stocking shelves with food, it seems like a regular job. If we describe the impact of how a food pantry can improve an individual's life and create more food justice, it has a different meaning. When we describe how food banks and food pantries can reduce health disparities, promote equity, and build bridges out of poverty, it will invite younger generations to become involved. This is why it is so important to move from outputs to outcomes—to describe not just the millions of pounds of food we provide but how an individual was able to take care of herself and her family because of the pantry.

When we describe how food banks and food pantries can reduce health disparities, promote equity, and build bridges out of poverty, it will invite younger generations to become involved.

Duplication of Services

One of Foodshare's new partner program coordinators, Yahaira Escribano, grew up in Hartford, Connecticut. She said, "Very quickly I realized that Foodshare has way too many small pantries that are open one to two times a month. I felt my time wasn't being used effectively because with so many pantries, most of which are small, it is a challenge to designate extra time and support to help elevate agencies to the next level so they become more sustainable and offer more services." Hartford is seventeen square miles and has fifty food pantries. That's a lot. And this is not including community kitchens and shelters.

Part of this can be explained by the fact that Hartford has a high poverty rate of 31 percent (in 2018) and a need for free food. But this is all the more reason to provide coordinated, holistic services to make it easier for people to receive food assistance and other support. Yahaira described, "I and so many others believe that a stronger coordination between these smaller agencies can have a profound, positive impact with the services they provide; and not just food either."

Even before COVID-19, the mayor's office was supportive of consolidating food pantries in the city of Hartford, recognizing that it doesn't help residents to have many small groups working in silos. We diffuse our resources with splintered groups. We lose our impact by having many small pantries working in isolation. At the onset of COVID-19, recognizing that more people would need food, part of the early emergency response was to identify food pantry locations and their hours of operation. Despite having many food programs, the pandemic exposed that many of them are open only a few hours each month. Data and information can be really powerful to drive changes. Yahaira said, "It wasn't until COVID-19 that the gaps and resilience in our emergency food system were more clearly revealed. That said, this is a moment to be creative and take risks, to take steps towards a more holistic and impenetrable network."

Yahaira led a working group on food security for the city of Hartford to provide recommendations for the mayor's office. She believes that the city can play a strong leadership role in helping to consolidate food pantries. Ideally, this would include a collaborative effort between the city and Foodshare, partnering with the Hartford Foundation for Public Giving, to provide incentives for food pantries to merge. For example, small grants (around $4,000) could be awarded to help agencies or churches partner and renovate their space. Foodshare could incentivize groups to merge by providing food credits and small grants for equipment and refrigerators. Let's explore why this makes sense.

Consolidation of Smaller Pantries

For years at Foodshare, and I'll bet this is true for many other food banks, if an organization wanted to become a member of the food bank, they were approved as long as they met some basic requirements. The result is that over the course of thirty-five years, we have developed a hodgepodge group of food pantries that vary in scope, size, operations, missions, and values. As a Feeding America member, we are required to conduct site visits with all food pantries and meal programs at least once every two years. Lower-capacity pantries often have challenges completing paperwork and require more staff involvement. The result is that staff spend more time with pantries that are providing fewer services in the community.

The result is that over the course of thirty-five years, we have developed a hodgepodge group of food pantries that vary in scope, size, operations, missions, and values.

While food bank staff will still need to document compliance (making sure pantries submit monthly paperwork and maintain food safety regulations), we want to ensure they have time to support capacity building (making sure pantries are using best practices). Foodshare started adding additional requirements to our membership agreement, such as requiring pantries to be open more than twice per month, paying attention to geography so that a new pantry cannot open if there is another pantry within the same neighborhood, and making sure that a pantry is collaborating with other local programs. Here are some ideas to create stronger, more holistic pantries.

Food banks can identify low-capacity pantries. By this I mean pantries that

- Have limited hours and days of operation;
- Do not have paid staff;
- Do not offer client choice;
- Do not provide fresh produce or other perishables;
- Do not provide referrals or other wraparound services;
- Have long wait times with people waiting outside;
- Do not have a mission statement;

- Add unnecessary burdens for people to receive food (such as proof of poverty);
- Do not partner with other community organizations in their area; and
- Are not interested or willing to try new approaches.

Food banks can work with these pantries to

1. Build their capacity to adopt best practices (i.e., provide trainings and support over the course of a year), especially if there are no other pantries nearby,
2. Merge or consolidate several smaller pantries located close together to create more holistic pantries, and
3. Eliminate some pantries from the network if they are not willing or able to make changes.

I know, this may not seem like a very popular sentiment. It seems counterintuitive to remove pantries when a lot of people are in need. Not everyone is going to like it. But this is the necessary step if we truly want to reinvent food pantries. The result will be that food banks will spend more energy and resources to support pantries that are willing and able to promote long-term health, stability, and financial well-being.

It is human nature to be territorial, whether as part of a church or a nonprofit agency, because people become attached to their individual programs, congregations, and volunteers. How do we encourage them to merge with another church or pantry? It requires relationships, trust, leadership, and a shift in perspective. Data can help. Food banks can start by gathering information about their food pantry network, map out the locations and hours of operation to identify obvious gaps and duplication of services. Measuring the capacity of pantries can help, not just by the pounds of food they order but on other best practices. Identify the low-capacity pantries.

Fitting with a key theme you've no doubt noticed throughout this book, there isn't one way to consolidate and merge pantries. I'm not proposing a cookie-cutter or one-size-fits-all approach. But I am proposing a paradigm shift and a new vision. It will look different in each community because the agencies, stakeholders, and leaders will be different. Consolidating pantries can create economies of scale by merging resources of food, volunteers, space, and talent. This will

Consolidating pantries can create economies of scale by merging resources of food, volunteers, space, and talent. This will help create more holistic pantries.

help create more holistic pantries. Where gaps exist and there are no food programs available, food banks can partner with existing anchor organizations such as clinics, community service agencies, libraries, and schools to create an on-site pantry or mobile program.

Reducing the overall number of pantries will help food bank staff to devote their time and resources to support pantries that align with the food bank's mission and vision for the future. However, it is important to point out that nonprofit or faith-based organizations that run food pantries are sovereign and autonomous agencies. A food bank does not have the authority to force them to merge with another agency. This is why it's important to provide a compelling case for how merging resources will benefit the people in the community—our ultimate goal.

Community Food Hubs

As important as it is to identify low-capacity pantries, it is equally important to identify the super pantries, the rock stars, and the model programs that already exist in the network. Food banks can use this information to allocate resources to help the higher-capacity pantries serve as community food hubs. Throughout the book, I have provided tools and new strategies for building food security. I have encouraged you to take one step. You may choose to try one of these approaches. That's great! And if you're ready for more, here is the whole toolbox. The vision of creating community food hubs that provide a one-stop-shopping hand up instead of many small pantries offering handouts. This is where all of the tools come together. Ready?

Imagine a coordinated, holistic approach to hunger in your community. Envision a group of robust pantries that serve as community food hubs that are available geographically throughout the region. They are open several days a week with some evening and weekend hours and staffed with full-time employees paid living wages with benefits.

Community food hubs will be well publicized so people know where they are located and when they are open. Guests won't feel embarrassed to go get help. These holistic food pantries will be designed like small groceries to offer full client choice with healthy perishable and non-perishable food and other household necessities. The community food hubs will provide more than food; they will create opportunities for individuals to build skills and work toward goals with on-site classes and workshops. They will have resource centers to provide access to computers and referrals to additional programs. Trained coaches will motivate individuals to work on goals and will help guests enroll in federal food assistance programs and community programs to address the root causes of hunger.

Community food hubs will provide welcoming and empowering spaces for guests to network, build social capital, and advocate for bigger systems and policy changes. People will come for food, but they will also come for community and a sense of belonging. There will be opportunities for guests to raise their voices about their experience with food insecurity and to help develop long-term solutions. The community food hubs will be part of the social safety net, and therefore the government (starting with municipalities, then state, then federal) will help fund the food hubs to provide food and wraparound services to help people get back on their feet.

Logically, many of the food hubs within a food bank network will evolve from existing food pantries that are already strong model programs. We don't have to start from scratch. Resources can be allocated to support the holistic food hubs. By consolidating and merging several smaller pantries, you will also have ancillary pantries throughout the community to make it easier for people to seek help. I am not advocating for only community food hubs with no other food pantry programs. If there are towns or locations without an existing strong pantry, the food bank can work with an existing social service program or anchor organization to add a healthy food pantry component.

These community food hubs will work closely with other agencies and antipoverty programs and won't operate in isolation. They will complement but not duplicate other agencies, and they will support one another with joint fundraising opportunities. Close your eyes for a minute and really let this sink in. Imagine what this would look like in your local area. Feels good, right?

Leadership and Enforcement

Creating community food hubs will take coordination, planning, communication, and coalition building. It may take some matchmaking. And you guessed it, it takes time, trust, and relationships. I'm not talking about a hostile takeover but rather a coordinated effort. This is not something you want to do lightly or quickly. First it requires a strong commitment and clear statement of why consolidation of pantries and creation of holistic food hubs will benefit the community. This should come first from the CEO of the food bank and can be echoed and reinforced by other influential and well-respected community leaders. Obviously, you'll need to engage your board of directors and hopefully they can be strong cheerleaders for the change. Who else can you invite to help shift the paradigm? Mayors, physicians, CEOs, religious leaders, maybe a sports icon. You will want to find key individuals and community groups who can speak about the new vision and paradigm shift. These are the early adopters and champions who will help bring others on board.

As a food bank, once you've decided to consolidate programs and create food hubs, start talking about it. You can describe the broad vision for your network to create holistic community food hubs in routine emails to your network, as part of compliance visits, and as part of an agency summit or annual conference for all food pantries. Plant the seeds early. You don't want to blindside people, and you want them to feel part of the movement. When you describe a potential merger for specific pantries, they can help design the changes for themselves.

You can also focus on one region at a time. You don't have to tackle your whole network all at once. Once you identify an area that is ripe for consolidation, the food bank can host small group meetings in that neighborhood (preferably not at the food bank) with key pantries and other community groups to show the vision, hear concerns, and strategize a plan.

Consolidation will require both a carrot and a stick to persuade pantries to collaborate. Food banks can encourage smaller pantries located close together to merge with the "carrot" of small grants, food credits, trainings, and additional volunteers, with support from local corporations or foundations. Food banks can enforce the mergers with the "stick" of new regulations within a specific time frame, say one year, or the pantries will not be able to renew their membership and receive food and resources from the food bank. Make a plan with a time line for staging in these changes, even if done over several years. If done thoughtfully and in partnership with community leaders, this can be a win-win situation. If done behind closed doors with little communication to your network and as a top-down edict, it can burn a lot of bridges.

Again, relationships are key. Yahaira from Foodshare has been working closely with agencies in Hartford for the past year, and she can see the progress taking shape. She describes, "More pantries are collaborating with each other and with other non-food community organizations. I've been able to connect agencies and have more programs work together and not create new ones."

Be prepared for resistance from some community members, and you may find resistance from some food bank staff too. The traditional role of food banks is to provide more food in the community, so some will argue that reducing agencies goes against the food bank mission. But remember, we have been providing billions of pounds of food over decades, yet food insecurity remains a persistent problem. We can do better. We can aim higher. It is time to evolve to more holistic and coordinated networks that comprehensively serve our communities.

There is often resistance to change, and fear of losing ownership of an individual program. As part of a merger or consolidation, encourage the pantry coordinators to rename or rebrand the food pantry program to reflect the new "blended family."

Strategies to reduce resistance to consolidation include the following:

- Create a clear vision and direction for your network.
- Provide frequent and open communication about potential changes.
- Use data and map the network to identify gaps, duplications, low- and high-capacity pantries.
- Create new guidelines and a realistic time line to build the capacity of the network.
- Provide incentives for community food hubs and also restrictions if smaller programs don't comply.

- Host roundtable discussions with food pantries and other community groups to encourage feedback.
- Recognize food pantries as experts in the community.
- Foster creativity to create more holistic programs.

Learning Opportunities

Another great way to build community buy-in, and develop a grassroots movement to coordinate food pantry services is to create opportunities for food pantries to network and learn from one another. An annual conference or agency summit presents a strong opportunity to share best practices with the whole network.

You can also host regional roundtable discussions that are held at high-capacity pantries and anchor institutions. This shouldn't be seen as a presentation from the food bank but rather an opportunity for local programs to network and share their best practices and lessons learned. The food bank can facilitate the meeting and provide some structure, but the main agenda item is peer-to-peer learning.

The Hartford Foundation for Public Giving occasionally hosts bus tours to highlight community programs that are doing great work for potential donors. The foundation invites local financial donors to meet at a designated location, load onto a bus, and, as a group, visit three or four community sites. As a food bank, can you host this type of bus tour with pantries in your network? Talk with a local corporation about underwriting the expenses. Either as part of this tour or as a separate tour, you could invite potential new community partners, funders, and researchers to visit these same locations to help build the vision of community food hubs.

It can also be beneficial for food bank staff who are not primarily responsible for agency relations to see various food pantries in your community. Remember, when you've seen one food pantry, you've seen one food pantry. If we want to create a coordinated network of high-capacity pantries that utilize best practices, it's important for various stakeholders, including food bank staff, to see in real life what that can look like.

The future is bright! New partners, new leaders, and a vision for community food hubs can help us truly reinvent our charitable food network.

Action Steps

- Start building relationships with health-care providers such as health clinics and hospitals to offer food as medicine.
- Talk with local colleges and universities about student hunger and develop appropriate strategies based on resources.
- As a food bank, gather data about the food pantries in your network to identify low- and high-capacity agencies.
- Create a plan for supporting, consolidating, or eliminating low-capacity pantries within a specified time frame.
- Develop a vision for a comprehensive, coordinated system of community food hubs for your region.
- Identify champions and cheerleaders who can support your vision.
- Host conferences, roundtable discussions, or bus tours whereby food pantry staff and other key stakeholders can network and share best practices.

Your actions matter. The steps you take can make a huge, positive impact in your community.

Resources

Boston Medical Center. "Preventive Food Pantry." https://www.bmc.org/nourishing
-our-community/preventive-food-pantry.

Community Food Centres Canada. https://cfccanada.ca/en/Home.

Feeding America, "Addressing Food Insecurity among College Students." 2019.
https://www.feedingamerica.org/sites/default/files/2019-10/College%20
Hunger%20Landscape%20-%20Brief.pdf.

Food Research & Action Center. "Screen & Intervene." https://www.frac.org
/screen-intervene.

Geisinger Fresh Food Farmacy. https://www.geisinger.org/freshfoodfarmacy.

Long, Christopher, Brett Rowland, Susan Steelman, and Pearl McElfish. "Outcomes of Disease Prevention and Management Interventions in Food Pantries
and Food Banks: A Scoping Review," *BMJ Open* 9, no. 8 (2019): e029236.
https://doi.org/10.1136/bmjopen-2019-029236.

CHAPTER 13

Conclusion: Take One Step

Imagine that it is 1982. The top movie is *E.T.*, and A Flock of Seagulls is playing on the radio. I know, some of you weren't born yet, but use your imagination. The country is in an economic recession, and the federal government just cut the food stamp budget. After church one Sunday a woman tells another parishioner that her husband lost his job and they are having a tough time buying groceries. Several members of the church decide to do something to help. They hold a community meeting and invite members of the church and several other community organizations, social service agencies, and government officials to brainstorm about what to do. They form a committee to design a community-based program that can serve as a stepping stone to help people get back on their feet.

They identify a convenient location in the middle of town, close to the church and on a bus line, where space is available. The program is created as a hub for basic needs, community services, job training, and wraparound supports. There are meeting rooms for classes and individualized coaching sessions and also a large community space for gatherings. The group partners with local companies, community organizations, and government agencies to offer programs under one roof to provide a convenient one-stop shopping experience. Oh yeah, and they provide food. They set up a pantry where people can choose their food like a grocery store. The program is designed so people can come for food, enroll in benefits, take classes, work on soft skills, apply for jobs, meet neighbors, and advocate for community changes.

The group wants to make sure that people know about the new program, so they advertise it in local newspapers and radio stations to raise awareness. People who receive services speak up about their situations and are invited to speak at town meetings and to testify before the state legislature. Their advocacy prompts changes to state safety net programs, including additional funding to support basic needs. A nonprofit organization runs the program, but the city government and local corporations provide funding to support the bottom line. People who have benefited from the program come back and work as staff. The program becomes an anchor institution where people come to receive help for a short period of time, build stability, and bounce back. Across town, another coalition forms to create a sister program, but there isn't a need for multiple small agencies providing the same service.

A Different Scenario of How the System Evolved

If this utopian vision had come to pass, imagine where we might be today. With coordination at the local level to provide comprehensive services, there wouldn't be a need for multiple small agencies handing out food. With community food hubs that were open throughout the week, there wouldn't be a need for people to wait in long lines. This would reduce the amount of stigma and embarrassment associated with seeking help. The role of food banks would have been to serve as a warehouse to collect and distribute food regionally but also to serve as a clearinghouse for resources, research, and activism. They would have advocated for federal food assistance programs and a strong government safety net. Cuts to food stamps and child nutrition programs in the early 1980s might have been reversed.

Because the community food hubs were new programs, maybe the food bank would have partnered with a local university to carefully evaluate them to identify which services were most effective. Food banks would use the data to scale evidence-based programs throughout the various hubs and would continuously gather data to share what worked with other food banks. If food banks had evolved differently, they might have standardized services, such as client choice, within the hubs and within the national network. Food banks might have trained volunteers to serve as allies for equity to build social capital. Maybe they would have hired community organizers or community health workers to identify marginalized populations and underserved communities to make sure they were aware of the food hubs and used their services. This might have reduced health disparities.

The food banks and food hubs would have been public–private partnerships from the beginning. Since they would have coordinated with other government programs, social service agencies, and antipoverty organizations, they might have increased financial well-being and reduced poverty for people seeking help, which in turn would have reduced food insecurity. Maybe they could have reversed the widening gap in income inequality that began in the 1970s. Maybe, who knows?

Unfortunately, this is not how the system evolved. We have witnessed an unbelievable growth in the number of hunger-relief organizations around the country since the early 1980s, typically working independently and tirelessly, yet food insecurity remains a stubborn public health problem that affects millions of Americans.

We can't rewind our history, but we can learn from it. We can make changes now. What will the future look like? Fortunately, we don't need to start from scratch. Let's lean into the amazingly robust, well-respected, and strong network of food banks and food pantries nationwide. As a

I'm not advocating that we close our doors, but let's start changing our business as usual.

network, we can leverage our incredible collective energy and power to end hunger. Let's remember that no one thought that food banks would be a long-term solution to hunger. Food bank staff often claim that we want to put ourselves out of business. I'm not advocating that we close our doors, but let's start changing our business as usual. The tools in this book can help to reinvent our existing programs to be a bridge, catalyst, springboard, and a launch pad to stability, health, equity, food security, justice, and well-being.

I am inspired by the many agencies that have adjusted with the times. There are food pantries embedded in anchor organizations that operate like the vision I just described. Innovative food pantries are providing cooking classes, offering case management and job training, and providing wraparound services to boost food security and self-sufficiency. Food pantries are combatting chronic diseases with diabetes prevention programs. Progressive food banks are setting wellness policies and promoting social justice. Canada has a national model of community food centers that offer healthy, nutritious food in a dignified manner, with services that promote civic engagement and empowerment. How similar or different are the local food pantries in your community to these examples? What changes would you like to make?

Think about how much time your organization spends "downstream" focused on immediate food needs—collecting, distributing, trucking, sorting, bagging, and handing out food—versus how much time you spend focused "upstream" on why people need help affording food—finding ways to prevent individuals from becoming food insecure in the first place, advocating for safety net programs, and empowering individuals to set and reach goals. It's time to commit and invest in longer-term solutions that shift from emergency to empowerment.

The charitable food system cannot solve the problem of hunger alone. We are one piece of the puzzle. Government at various levels (local, state, and federal) also needs to be a key ally and stakeholder as part of the equation to end hunger. We need politicians to secure funding for SNAP, increase the minimum wage, and make health care affordable. We need top-down federal policy changes. We need corporations to do their part too by paying living wages and providing benefits to reduce wage disparity between executives and their employees. And (not but) we need grassroots, bottom-up, community-based changes to help people help themselves. The overall goal is not only to meet the immediate need for food but to stop the cycle of hunger and poverty for the next generation. How do we create this paradigm shift? Where do we start?

There isn't one silver bullet to end hunger. But there are many ways, big and small, that you can begin to make changes in your community today. Please don't get intimidated. Just get started.

Menu of Options

There isn't one silver bullet to end hunger. But there are many ways, big and small, that you can begin to make changes in your community today. Please don't get intimidated. Just get started.

Each chapter in this book describes best practices and provides tangible examples with action steps. Think of these topics as items on a menu. Maybe you just want to start with an appetizer, like painting the walls in your food pantry a bright color or changing the language you use in your newsletters to describe hunger in a more strength-based way focusing on social justice. If you're selecting an entrée, maybe you're ready to train volunteers to provide referrals to local community programs or to allow guests to choose their food with dignity. If you're ready for a dessert, maybe you want to use the SWAP system to rank food nutritionally to increase the supply and demand for healthy food. As you choose different menu options, you'll want to add your own special sauce, your unique twist on providing charitable food that reflects your local community needs, resources, and the diverse populations that you serve.

And if you're really ready, you can order the whole enchilada! You can create a holistic community food hub that provides healthy food, an empowering space to build social capital, and wraparound services. This menu option is best shared in collaboration with other community groups to build collective impact. This food hub will create opportunities for people to network and advocate and foster a sense of belonging.

As a food bank, you can help build the capacity of your food pantry network to try these menu options. Discuss these best practices in routine emails and in annual conferences, provide trainings and small grants, and help pantries network with one another. As a food pantry, talk with your staff and volunteers about the options you'd like to try that will make a difference for your guests.

Yes, millions of people are hungry in America, but they are hungry for more than just food. They are hungry for social connection, community, and justice. And this requires time to build relationships and trust between staff, volunteers, guests, and other community members. It requires space to gather and share stories. It requires patience to try new things and mess up and try again. It takes courage to get out of our comfort zones.

Traditional food pantries pride themselves on efficiency—moving food as quickly as possible to as many people as possible. Community food hubs will look less like a well-oiled machine. They will involve more time to interact and build relationships. They may look messier when you involve more community organizations. They may be a little more chaotic when you blur the lines between volunteers and guests. The calendar may be more hectic when you host events and workshops with other organizations. But community food hubs will have a more sustainable impact on the people they serve. They will also be more vibrant and joyous because they will not just fill bellies but will help fill the soul.

I hope that this book will spur you to action to apply some of these tools and evidence-based practices into the work you do. I hope you feel inspired and motivated to move FROM

- Emergency TO empowerment;
- Scarcity mentality TO abundance mindset;
- Sympathy TO empathy;
- Pounds of food TO nutritional quality of food;
- Embarrassment TO engagement;
- Communication TO collaboration;
- Compliance TO capacity building;
- Outputs TO outcomes;
- Short-term Band-Aid TO stability and self-sufficiency; and
- Transaction TO transformation.

Opportunities for New Funders

You may be thinking, these ideas sound good, but how in the heck are we going to pay for them? I hear you, but think about this. Increasingly, funders want to see collaboration among community groups, and they want to ensure that several organizations are working together to tackle difficult

Unfortunately, competition among nonprofit organizations holds us back from true transformational growth.

social problems rather than working alone. Unfortunately, competition among nonprofit organizations holds us back from true transformational growth. Collaboration will open the door to new and bigger funding sources. Offering new programs and changing your status quo can be an invitation for new funding partners.

This may require some vulnerability. When we acknowledge that the people we serve will be better when we collaborate with others, we need to be brave enough to let go of organizational egos and trust that there will be enough funding and resources to support our good work. This requires a gut check. Be honest and clear about the strengths and limitations of each organization. Your nonprofit might be best suited to serve as the leader for one project, while another agency in the community may be better suited to lead another project. Your organization may receive grant funding for one project, and another nonprofit or social service provider may receive funding for a separate project. Include one another as subcontractors. Write letters of support for one another. Serve on advisory councils together.

Changing the conversation about hunger means measuring our success not just by how many pounds of food we distribute, but what type of effect we have had on the health, financial well-being, and long-term food security of the people we serve. This is hard work! And we can't do it alone. Funders want to see outcomes and to know that their dollars are making an impact. We will have better outcomes and bigger impacts (meaning there will be more people who are food secure and thriving) when we partner with others.

As we create community food hubs that promote health, food security, and financial well-being, there is a great opportunity to conduct research to document that they work. Talk with Feeding America's terrific research team about opportunities to conduct research, contact university researchers who are interested in food security, and check out materials in the resource section at the end of chapter 9. As we build evidence that community food hubs are effective at promoting long-term food security, it will provide incentives for city, state, and federal governments, and also corporations and philanthropic foundations, to provide funding. Data is powerful.

Organizational Readiness for Change

We're doing a lot of good work, sometimes really amazing, awe-inspiring, great work. But we can do better. It's important to get organizational buy-in and commitment to prepare for change.

Think about the types of changes you want to make and who will be responsible for making the changes happen. Think about the various staff members and departments within your food bank or food pantry. It helps if they understand *why* the changes are important before you describe what will change and how and when. You'll want to engage as many stakeholders as possible. Many of the changes we're talking about here are a paradigm shift from your routine activities, so you really need buy-in from staff, guests, donors, board members, and volunteers.

Changing attitudes and mindsets is just the start. Following through with actions and holding your organization accountable is another big step.

Changing attitudes and mindsets is just the start. Following through with actions and holding your organization accountable is another big step. Here are ten steps for getting organizational buy-in and creating change within your organization:

1. Talk about the change you want to make and ask for feedback. Listen to concerns and opinions. Brainstorm and build your pitch for change. Get commitment from leadership and describe the proposed changes at staff meetings and board retreats.

2. Visit other organizations who have incorporated the change you want to make to see it in action. Collaborate with other community organizations such as social service providers, universities, health-care providers, or advocacy organizations so you can pool resources.

3. Spell out the changes in your yearly operating plan. Include smart goals to hold staff accountable to make the changes happen. Use data to provide some metrics for where you want to be a year from now. Start with a pilot program and grow the program over time.

4. Provide trainings for staff and volunteers about the values and vision that support the change (the "why"), along with a clear plan to implement the change (the "what").

5. Write about your new programs or the new way of operating in your newsletters, e-appeals, and annual reports to let your supporters know what you're doing. Include quotes and photos from people who participate and benefit from the program to show the impact.

6. Be prepared that you may lose some volunteers or staff along the way who don't appreciate your new vision. Remember, this is not always easy but is often necessary to stay true to our mission and values. You will gain new volunteers along the way who hear about your new programs. This can lead to new community partners.

7. Fund-raise for your new programs. Money talks and will help you build greater buy-in within your organization. Describe your new initiatives with existing funders and seek out new funders—talk with local community foundations and corporations to describe your new vision and ask for their support for more holistic programming. Funders will want to know that you are partnering with other organizations, so by collaborating with others you increase your chances of funding. Do you see the domino effect here? Cool, right?

8. Formalize and codify the changes through written policies and procedures, for example in your mission statement, nutrition policy, or equity statement.

9. As you revamp existing programs to match your new vision, consider a new name or a new logo. This isn't just window dressing. Remember, words have power.

10. Evaluate how you're doing. Keep an open mind and examine what is working and not working. This will provide continuous learning and lead you back to #1 above when you want to revise the program or start a new one.

Big, Hairy, Audacious Goals

Several years ago, Gloria McAdam, the CEO of Foodshare for thirty years, was inspired by Jim Collins's book *Built to Last*, in which he describes big, hairy, audacious goals. Gloria was a visionary, and she encouraged Foodshare not just to set yearly goals but to set big and hairy goals in audacious ways. Sadly, Gloria lost her battle with cancer in 2019. To recognize her contributions, Foodshare dedicated our building in her honor. When you walk into Foodshare, there is a plaque with Gloria's picture on it to honor her memory and the great work she did to fight hunger in Greater Hartford.

This book is all about big, hairy, audacious goals. It's about reinventing the way we conduct business. It's about not being afraid to try new things with trial and error, to continuously learn and fail forward. It's about using data and evidence to inform our work using best practices and sharing these ideas with others. It's about building new creative partnerships and getting out of our comfort zones. I think Gloria would be excited about the big, hairy, and audacious goals we can achieve as we reinvent the charitable food system.

During COVID-19, Feeding America described how "the charitable food assistance network remains strong and resilient. Our national network is getting creative and innovating to respond to the health crisis. This shows how nimble, flexible, and prepared we are to take on new challenges." We couldn't sit back and say, "this is how it has always been done," or "this is how we've always done things." The status quo wasn't an option. We all had to pivot, to innovate, to change up our routines. We rose to the occasion. We transformed the way we did our day-to-day operations to respond to the increased need for food while protecting public health.

Change is possible! We are fully capable of adjusting and evolving. When we embrace the idea of reinvention, we stay nimble and flexible, we continue to listen and learn, to evolve. Thomas Edison described how he invented the lightbulb by saying, "I haven't failed. I've just found 10,000 ways that won't work."

> *When we embrace the idea of reinvention, we stay nimble and flexible, we continue to listen and learn, to evolve.*

In the book *You Are a Badass*, Jen Sincero encourages readers to get clear on what they want, and she provides advice and motivation for how to go after your dreams. At the end of the book she describes a low point in her life where she began questioning her own beliefs and suggestions. Then she decided to take her own advice, live by her own mantras, and practice what she preached. Spoiler alert, it worked out. My favorite line in the book is when she says, "This. Shit. Works."

I have argued for reinventing our charitable food system. No easy feat. I recommend bold changes and a paradigm shift away from the status quo. Here's what I have found. When food pantries offer choice, guests and volunteers appreciate it and there is less food waste. When food banks use the SWAP stoplight system, they order healthier food. When food pantry guests volunteer their time, they feel empowered.

When food pantries provide fresh produce and nutritional nudges, guests select healthier food. When food pantries offer coaching, members are more self-sufficient and food secure. When we ask people to share their experiences dealing with hunger, they appreciate someone listening to them and they feel seen. When we gather data about our programs, it helps prompt changes that improve the work we do. When food banks partner with other community organizations, we are stronger together. Believe me, this shit works!

Maybe your food bank or food pantry is approaching your fortieth anniversary, or maybe only its first anniversary. Either way, now is the perfect time to examine the way you operate. Maybe you're opening a brand new pantry and are looking for ideas for how to start. You can incorporate best practices right from the beginning. We have the resources, ingenuity, and brainpower to send satellites around the planet, to create self-driving cars, and to print three-dimensional objects from digital files, and yet millions of Americans do not have access to enough food. We can do better.

I hope that by reading this book you have had some aha moments and are thinking differently about how we can address hunger in our local communities. I hope this book will help change how we describe the problem of hunger and attitudes about what types of programs are most effective. I want to hear about your lightbulb moments and the steps you've taken to reinvent the charitable food system in your community. I'd love to hear about your experiences and solutions you've tried so I can learn and share them with others.

Dream a Little (or a Lot) Bigger

My colleague Erica Greeley is the vice president of economic mobility at Feeding America. She leads the strategy to help working families achieve food security. During a recent conference, she told a very compelling story, and with her permission I am retelling it for your benefit.

Erica was born and grew up in Kenya. Years later she returned to visit Lydia, a family friend, who lived in the foothills of Mount Kenya. It was a cloudy day, and Erica described her disappointment at not being able to see the mountain. Lydia looked quizzically at Erica and asked what she meant that she couldn't see the mountain. Erica pointed to the clouds covering up the mountain, which seemed obvious to her, and she wondered if her friend might have misunderstood her. Lydia gave a wise and knowing look back to Erica, pointed higher above the clouds, and aimed at the top of the mountain. She told Erica that she wasn't looking high enough.

The moral of the story, Erica said, is that we all need to look higher and dream bigger. When we get stuck in the status quo of "feeding the hungry" and "meeting the need," we will stare directly into thick clouds. It will be hard to see a new direction. But by looking outside our comfort zones, aiming higher than we have previously dreamed, we will see new solutions.

We have the ability to dramatically change the way we provide charitable food. To reinvent the charitable food system to foster health, social justice, and long-term food security. I don't have all the answers, and there is certainly no silver bullet, but I know for sure that we can do better. Don't settle for the way we've always done things. Innovate, ask hard questions, try new things, don't be afraid to fail, and share your story with others. Are you ready? Take one step.

Action Steps

- Make a commitment, a pledge, an intention to take at least one action step outlined in this book.
- Write it down and, most importantly, talk about it with others in your community. Your words have power.
- As Mahatma Ghandi said, "Be the change you want to see in the world."
- Go ahead, aim higher and dream bigger.

About the Author

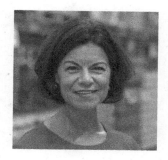

Katie S. Martin is the executive director of the Foodshare Institute for Hunger Research & Solutions. She is recognized as a thought leader on food security issues. She earned a doctorate in Nutritional Science and Policy from Tufts University. Katie lives in Simsbury, Connecticut, is happily married to Chris Drew, is the proud mom of Carson and Brian, and is blessed to be the host mom for Kenny Aruwajoye from Nigeria. This is Katie's first book.